LIVE

SURVIVING A TERMINAL CANCER DIAGNOSIS

BOB ABBOTT

ABBOTT BOOKS

Library and Archives Canada Cataloguing in Publication.

Abbott, Robert
Live: Surviving a Terminal Cancer Diagnosis / Robert Abbott

(Live: Surviving a Terminal Cancer Diagnosis ; paperback)
ISBN 978-1-7380480-0-7

First Edition, December 2023

Dedicated to those starting their journey
and to those helping along the way.
Stay Strong.

AUTHOR'S NOTE

Everything in this book is true. I was given six months to live. I was devastated and scared beyond belief. I felt as if I had entered another dimension. Nothing seemed real. My voice had lost its strength. My eyes were empty. Despair and fear had taken over my life. My wife Darlene and my sons Bobby and Josh gave me back the will to live, the will to fight. The courage to search for and hold on to hope. When I accepted death I began to feel life again. That's when the fight to survive began.

PREFACE

It's been ten years since that horrific day in January 2014 when I received the final verdict no one is ever prepared to hear. At fifty-seven years old I'm told I have terminal cancer with at most six months to live. I'm to go home and get my affairs in order.

I fought against the odds and survived when others didn't. Today, though healthy, and active, there are times I can't sleep. When I do, I wake up sweating from the terrible dreams in which I'm reliving the nightmare I went through. I wonder if I'm losing my mind. Is death coming for me? Strangely enough, after everything I've been through, I think maybe that's okay. Have I made a difference in this world? Why did I survive when all the odds were stacked against me? Surgeons deal with the physical pain but no one offers you help for the psychological pain.

I feel guilty because I survived while so many others didn't. Why do I now feel my life doesn't matter? What impact have I had on this world? These questions continued to haunt me and made me feel lost to the point I was uncertain about a happy, fulfilling life. My wife suggested that I write down my experiences during this journey. She felt that even if I help one person navigate their journey with hope and determination, then perhaps that is the reason for my survival and my reason to go on living.

My story will be mixed up, confusing, tragic, good, bad, and at times even amusing. I'll relate every emotion and sentiment which often overpowered me at the most inopportune times. My one wish is that it helps you in some way with your journey. The most important advice I can give is to never give up and to stay strong. Be assured there will be tough times ahead, dark moments when you want to give up because the struggle just seems too daunting. I know it will be difficult, but find a reason to get up each day, to want to fight, to want to live. My reason to fight to live was my wife and sons.

If I can survive a literal death sentence, so can you with the belief and hope that anything is possible. Fight with everything you have. Find the inner strength to go on. A strength you never imagined you had. With a strong attitude and a strong support system, it is possible to come back from a terminal illness. And if the worst happens, as it appeared to be the case many times in my struggle, I truly believed it is okay to die with respect and dignity. My feeling was and still is, as long as you fight you can still die with dignity. If you don't fight back the disease you're suffering from wins and you die on its terms not yours.

I can assure you battling a life threatening illness is not peaceful or easy. I ask myself what does dying peacefully really mean. Dying peacefully to me is knowing you fought with all you had to survive, at peace that you didn't give up. As someone who fought the fight against terrible odds, I repeat that you have to fight to survive. If you die fighting, doesn't that fight give you dignity? Doesn't that fight give you a chance to survive? Doesn't that fight give your family more respect for you? Doesn't that fight send a positive message to family and friends? I would rather fight than just give up!

During my struggle raw fear and panic were my ever-present companions. I couldn't hide from the fear. It followed me everywhere. I couldn't sleep. I would sit in the chair in our living room and picture my family going on with their lives without me. I'm happy for them but sad I won't be there to enjoy life with them. How will they cope? How is my journey affecting their lives, their hope, and their faith? My two sons were faced with the undeniable fact that their father had been given six months to live. What was going through their minds? I know how scared I was. How must they feel? How must my wife feel? The nights are the worst when you are alone with your thoughts. The fear of dying is overwhelming, but the idea of leaving those you love behind is unbearable. Your existence is measured in months not years. I would look in the mirror and I wouldn't recognize the hollow, lifeless eyes staring back at me.

In this book I talk about the support I received and most important of all, the will and courage to survive. I talk about the journey through the health care system. I talk about family support and what it means when you're at the lowest point in your life. I talk about how the disease affects those around you. I talk about the dread of what tomorrow will bring. I talk about waiting for test results. I talk about the search for hope, just that one thread of hope no matter how inconsequential it may seem to a healthy person.

I hope the following pages describing my journey gives you the strength and courage to begin your journey with the belief that the fight is worth it. Life is worth it. All anyone can expect is for you to do your best. Draw from your own inner strength. Allow family and loved ones to give you their strength and love. Ask for their help. Reach out to friends. Don't give up. Positive thinking will lift your spirits and those around you.

Use your own life experiences to gather the strength you need to begin the battle in life that you're facing. When all seems lost find that ray of hope that brings you back to the fight.

This is my journey an ordinary man's Journey of Hope, Journey of Survival. My sincere desire is that it helps you travel a more peaceful path. My goal is to give hope to all who are or will be burdened with a difficult life journey. My sincere wish is that it helps you. Here is my story.

1

LIFE BEFORE CANCER

My name is Robert Paul Abbott. I was born on April 8th, 1956. I can hardly remember my first five years of life but by age six it seems my brain and memory kicked in, so that's where I'll begin. I begin my story talking about my father, my mother and my siblings. Some parts of my early years may seem unimportant but I strongly believe these early experiences helped form me into the person I am today. These life experiences would give me the foundation to fight the hardest battle I would ever have to face in my life. These early life experiences turned me into a stubborn, fearless child with the mindset to overcome any obstacle thrown my way. I wanted to enjoy life and just have fun. I brought these values into my adult life. As you read my stories replace them with yours and find within them the strength to begin your fight.

I grew up in a poor yet friendly and tightly knit section of our city where most families lived from paycheck to paycheck. My family was no different. My father, Ron finished high school in June 1940, which was a rarity back then. He joined the army and immediately entered World

War II. He went overseas on July 16th, 1940 just days after his seventeenth birthday on July 13th, 1940. My father returned home five years later on August 31st, 1945, he was twenty-two years old. He never talked about his time at war. I'm sure they were difficult. He handled the trauma of war in his own way as most veterans did back in the 1940's.

After returning from the war my father had many job opportunities but chose to work with his friends as a long-shoreman. While working there he was involved in a number of dockside accidents. Safety wasn't a big issue back in the mid 1940's. One particular accident involved two tons of glass breaking free from its strapping and landing across my father's chest breaking all his ribs and collapsing both lungs. It was feared he wouldn't survive. Weeks later he was back at work. He had ten children to support. My father's determination to live and fight I believe was instilled in me.

My father passed away at fifty-six years old still working as a longshoreman. I was twenty-two years old when he died at work, the same age he was when he returned from WW2. I was at dockside waiting to pick him up when he dropped to the ground and died instantly of a massive heart attack. I along with my brothers identified his body at the morgue. I can still see him lying on the table with small rocks lodged in his forehead. His left arm hanging from the side of the table. The sight of my father lying there devastated me and is forever etched in my mind.

My mother, Alice, and my father met after he returned home from the war. They married in 1947. Over the next thirteen years they had ten children, five girls and five boys of which I am the youngest boy. My mother stayed at home and raised all ten children.

My mother was a beautiful patient woman. Like most of the families back when I grew up other close relatives resided in the same household. My father and mother, my nine siblings, me, my father's mother, my father's stepfather, my father's sister and her two sons, lived with us. All together seventeen people lived in one house with one bathroom. This living arrangement was difficult for all of us but more so for our mother. My mother navigated through all the intricacies of this living arrangement with great patience and dignity. Many times she would tell me that she hated this living arrangement but she had no choice but to make the most of it.

My mother instilled in me the meaning of family and that you sacrifice everything to keep your family together. She had to manage sixteen different personalities and she did it masterfully. My mother's organizing, negotiating, delegating, and human resource skills would set me on my journey into adulthood, marriage and fatherhood.

Living with sixteen people in one household I took every opportunity to escape the house when I could. I would spend many days just riding my bicycle around the city, meeting new people and finding new friendships.

I considered myself a normal child who enjoyed having fun. Although thinking back on my early years I will admit nothing frightened me. No activity seemed too dangerous. I loved to jump from rooftops into snowbanks. During the summer I often played on a building along the harbour front. My friends and I would shimmy along the edge of this building perilously close to the polluted water. We had no fear. Hey, we were six years old. Falling in and drowning never entered our minds.

By the time I was six, I'd been hit by passing cars on three different occasions while playing in our neighborhood. The first time I broke an arm, the second a wrist, and the third a leg. My brother witnessed the last accident.

Instead of letting him help me I ran away for the simple reason I didn't want to go to the hospital. I'd been there twice before and I wasn't going back. No one was going to put another cast on me! How I managed to run away on a broken leg is still a mystery to me. I threatened my brother with a rock if he tried to take me home. My father came across us arguing on his way home from work and realized I was injured. There was no debating with my dad. He picked me up and carried me to the hospital, which was a short distance from our home. The only person that could over-power my fear of the hospital had me in his arms.

Life to me was to be lived and that meant having fun no matter the risk. The first day of school would change all that. At least that's how I saw it. I went straight into Grade one as kindergarten didn't exist at the time. My mother walked me to school the first day and promised me a quarter if I found my own way home. Walking home alone at that age was quite normal for the times. Also, a quarter bought much, much more than it does today. I arrived home by following an older boy who lived on my street. I never did receive the money my mother promised me. Each time I asked for it she'd say she'd give it to me later. Later in life I often joked with my mother that she owed me thousands of dollars in interest on that quarter.

I found Grade one boring so I decided I'd had enough of school as it was interfering with my fun. Needless to say, I didn't tell anyone. My six-year old brain concocted a plan which I believed was masterly and foolproof. The idea was to skip school and go on the "pip" as it was called in those days. I'd drop off my books in my classroom then head for the nearby lumber yard where I spent the day swinging on the big boom that moved lumber around the yard. I would have been scared to death if my two sons had done such a thing at the age of six. I attended school two maybe three days per week. As I reflect back it still amazes me how the principal never did inform my parents about me missing school.

One day my older brother spotted me in the lumber yard. He ran after me in order to bring me back to school. As he chased me I noticed a police officer standing by the corner of the street. I ran up to the officer and told him a strange man was after me. He confronted my brother while I continued to flee laughing all the while at my brother's predicament. He explained the situation to the policeman who luckily enough believed him. He never caught me and I continued to skip classes. In late May another brother spotted me. This time as he chased me, I fell over a fence and broke my right wrist. I've never asked my brothers why they didn't tell my parents that I skipped school. Perhaps it's an unspoken code of silence between brothers or maybe they didn't realize just how much school I missed.

At the end of May a neighbor told my parents they'd seen me around the neighborhood during school hours. From that point on I was grounded and only permitted outside to attend school. I didn't mind as the academic year was almost at an end. Exams began mid-June. Yep, there were indeed final exams for Grade one. Exams which you had to pass if you were to move on to Grade two. As my right wrist was broken, I asked my teacher, a Roman Catholic nun, if she would write my answers down for me. She snapped at me saying I most likely wasn't going to pass anyway because of too many missed school days. Despite my handicap. I wrote my exams and passed every one with the exception of English in which I received forty-nine percent. Fifty was a passing grade. There was no way I'd be kept back for one silly mark so I started summer vacation believing I had successfully completed Grade one.

The following September I walked to school with my buddies. Assembled in the gymnasium, we each lined up as our names were called for Grade two. My name was never called! I asked the nun why? Once again, she responded in a sarcastic tone that she'd already informed my parents that I wouldn't be placed in Grade two. Why didn't my parents fight this nun's decision? It wasn't fair I had to repeat Grade one for one lousy mark. In retrospect, I really couldn't blame the nun or my parents for my situation, in reality I hadn't attended enough school days to advance.

My heart hit the floor at the news I would repeat Grade one. Devastation is a much more appropriate term. I decided that day nothing like this would ever happen to me again. My second year of Grade one consisted of three rows of Grade two students and one row of Grade one students. Five Grade one students in total. I guess that's all that failed Grade one. During the year I paid close attention to the material taught to both grades. I excelled in my second year in Grade one and Grade two the following year. I went on to complete high school often receiving top marks. The experience of repeating Grade one and the failure I experienced in the gymnasium stayed with me into adulthood. Although a traumatic event, it helped shape my determination to overcome any obstacle thrown my way.

I had four older brothers in school ahead of me and thus I was rarely bothered by the bigger and older kids. Being Catholic I went to an all boy's school. My years in school were not that difficult especially after my experience in Grade one. Grade five was memorable for me. I was doing fine academically but a few of the boys in my class were being bullied. I didn't feel it was right so I stepped in and stopped the abuse. Three of these boys would follow me everywhere. They would hang around me during lunch and even follow me if we went on a school outing. We even walked home together. We were in the same class in Grade six and the bulling continued until I stepped in again. We became good friends and one of them reappeared into my life in Grade nine, he would end up changing my life forever.

In Grade five my teacher seemed to always have it out for me. One day the class was misbehaving and he commented that we were behaving like little children. He decided that we all had to take our bathroom break together and when we did we had to hold hands on the way. I refused to do this and every time during bathroom break I was punished. The teacher would put my head under the chalk holder under the blackboard. He would them hit me on the backside with a stick. This would happen twice a day for two weeks until the teacher conceded and we didn't have to hold hands going to the washroom. I never did tell my parents this story.

Growing up with four brothers and five sisters wasn't easy. All ten of us slept in two rooms. Five boys in one room with two sets of bunk beds. The two oldest twins occupied one set while the remaining three boys occupied the other. I shared the top bunk with a brother (who later became a firefighter). If I moved while sleeping, he would kick me and tell me not to bend my legs. As a result, to this day I still sleep with rigidly straight legs. The middle brother slept alone in the bottom bunk. Four of my sisters occupied the second room. They constantly griped at each other, complaining one or the other was taking up too much room in the bed which caused many a sleepless night for everyone. The remaining sister spent the majority of the first eight years of her life in hospital due to an orthopedic condition and therefore missed out on those sleepless nights.

Despite these sleeping arrangements we had many good times. You can imagine growing up in a five-bedroom house with seventeen people. As the second youngest you get lost in the crowd. The adults and your older siblings never listened to your opinion. You could decide to be passive or you could find creative ways to have your voice and opinion heard. I chose to be heard and picked the wrong way. I misbehaved and at fourteen years old hung around with a few hard cases that I thought were friends. We did some shady things and I was lucky not to end up in jail. Some of those friends actually ended up in prison later on in life.

One day my father called me into the back room of our house. He gave me a choice, continue hanging out with this group of friends and end up in jail or change my friends. He understood because of my stubborn personality he couldn't demand this. I took his advice and searched out new friends. I still thank my father for his wise counsel. Simple conversations with someone you love and respect can some-times change your life forever. The conversation I had with my father that day was one of those conversations and I will remember it forever.

I had been a member of the local boys club since I was eight years old but had left the club at fourteen when I started hanging out with this group of friends. After the conversation with my father, I rejoined the Knights of Columbus boys club. I tried it for a while but I wasn't happy. I wanted to experience new friendships, so I decided to check out another boys club where I signed up for their summer camp. In mid-July I informed my parents that I was going to camp for twenty-one days. I packed my clothes in my father's army backpack, said goodbye and walked up to the boys club where we boarded the yellow bus for the four-hour drive to Camp Sherwood.

The first few days at camp were challenging as I was a complete stranger. When we arrived at camp we were assigned twenty boys to each barrack. The bed assignment was based on seniority and physical capability. The bigger you were the more you could intimidate the smaller ones to get what you wanted. Being the new kid I received the worst bed which meant I was situated next to the barrack door and bathroom. I was constantly awoken by a steady stream of boys coming and going. Camp life was rigid with a weekly point system. We learned to make our bed military style and ensure the barrack was spotless clean. If not, the barrack lost points. Every week the barrack with the most points was rewarded with a movie night or a trip to the local town.

We got up at seven in the morning, early for a fourteen year old, and were given a crate of food for the day. We collected firewood for the fire pit to cook our meals. I was especially good at finding blasty boughs (branches that had turned red from cut down trees) which burned the hottest thus producing faster cooked meals. As a reward I didn't have to cook. To be honest, most days I didn't cook because it took too long, keeping me from more fun activities. As a result, I often ate cold tinned beans or spaghetti. The other boys laughed at me while they enjoyed their hot cooked meal.

Within a week I'd made friends with my room mates with one exception. This particular boy was older and bigger than any of us and everyone was afraid of him. He was especially verbally and physically aggressive towards me. I tolerated this for three days before deciding I'd had enough and came up with a plan. I discovered he couldn't swim. When the opportunity presented itself, I pushed him into the deep end of the camp swimming pool. I jumped in and punched him while he struggled to stay afloat. I knew this was risky knowing there was a possibility there would be payback later. As I've stated, I'd had enough of his torment so I was willing to risk the consequences. To my surprise and profound relief he respected what I had done and we became good friends for the remainder of the camp. The other boys showed me respect for what I had done, though I wasn't sure it if was true respect or simply fear of me. Either way it made the rest of the eighteen days at camp much more enjoyable. At the end of camp we had all become good friends. Many of those friendships exist to this day.

I had many memories from camp that have stayed with me throughout the years. Mail call was always somewhat disheartening. Parents wrote weekly enquiring how their sons were doing. The head councillor stood in the back of his truck and called out the names of the boys who received a letter. I never did receive one, being the last one left standing there, I would silently walk back to the barrack and comfort myself with the fact that my parents were occupied with nine other children.

On the second Sunday in camp all the parents came for a visit. Once again I was the last boy standing in the field. I reasoned my parents weren't there as they didn't have a car.

One night I left camp without anyone's knowledge. I went to the local town where I joined in with a group of people having a beach barbeque and ate the best hotdogs. It was great fun. Sneaking back into the camp wasn't as easy as sneaking out. I got caught. My barrack lost all our points for that week. My room mates forced me to make all the beds in the barrack for the remainder of the week. Later that week we played a barrack-to-barrack soccer tournament. We made it to the final game where I scored the winning goal. The prize was a trip to the local town. I was proud to be able to repay the boys for the points we'd lost because of my antics.

Time passed quickly and at the end of the twenty one days the yellow bus showed up at camp and drove us back to the club. All the parents were waiting to pick up their sons. My parents weren't there so I walked home alone. I knew they loved me, but I was fourteen. It still hurt they hadn't come to pick me up.

During my time at camp I learned how to take care of myself. I learned how to stand up for myself. I taught myself how to fight. I forged many lasting friendships. My camp experience helped me develop into the person I am today. As much as I was disappointed and hurt at the time when my parents didn't write or visit, they did have a lot going on at home with nine other children. Through it all they did a great job raising me. I will always remember, love, and respect them for that.

The summer before I started Grade nine, I had just turned fifteen and was still searching for fun. I had found new friends on my father's advice. We were enjoying the summer but it was coming to an end. For some reason an old friend from the previous troubled group I had hung out with showed up. We hung around together one weekend. I'm not sure why I did this but I remembered the fun and excitement of that friendship. I forgot my father's advice and that weekend nearly ruined my life.

This friend slipped me a hit of acid, a hallucinogenic drug. I began to feel strange and he told me what he had done. I was furious at him but the acid had begun to take hold of me. I began to hallucinate. That night I saw things in my head that I can't describe. Street lights appeared to be chasing me. Things fell from the sky that I can't explain to this day. Voices appeared slurred and my friend's face would get long and narrow. I experienced thoughts, feelings and emotions that night that I can never explain and I hope I would never experience again. I thought I was going to die. I prayed to God if I got through this I would become a better person. Ten hours later I was back from that trip. This so called friend would years later end up in federal prison.

In Grade nine one of the boys I had protected in Grade five and six was once again in my class. We reconnected as friends. He really struggled with his school work, so I helped him as much as I could. His greatest difficulty was with Math, one of my favorite subjects. During our final Math exam in the gymnasium I realized he was having difficulty with the test. I finished my exam reached back and took his exam. I wrote his test and passed it back to him. I received 95% in my final, he got 60%. I remembered how I felt that September back in Grade one when I realized I had failed. He was a good friend, who was I hurting. I am sure it helped him as he later passed high school and went on to have a good life.

I tried to keep my promise to God to be a better person then came high school. During that summer before school I would have an encounter with the police. One weekend my friends and I were down in the valley, a local area where young people gathered to party. Everyone in the valley that night were either drunk or stoned. I preferred drinking at that time and I had too many for a sixteen year old. Suddenly the police showed up. Everyone ran, I was so intoxicated, I couldn't run if I wanted to.

The police caught me, handcuffed me and brought me to the police station. Without explanation I was stripped to my underwear and forcefully brought inside to the jail. I decided I wasn't going in there so I grabbed hold of the bars and refused to go in. The police officers proceeded to beat the crap out of me. They hit me everywhere except in my head. There were no cameras back then so they could do whatever they wanted. They eventually freed my hands and threw me into the cell. Every part of my body hurt. When I awoke that morning in the cell even my head hurt. I was released 7:00 a.m that morning. I had spent six hours lying in that horrible place. What a relief to walk out of the police station that morning. I walked home and my father greeted me at the front door. He asked where I had been all night. I told him I had slept at a friend's house and apologized for not phoning him.

I knew how much he worried so I had to lie as the truth would have hurt him. I covered up that night in jail and the beating the police had given me. As I lay in jail that night with just my underwear on the thought of becoming a lawyer entered my mind.

In high school, hockey was my favorite sport. I tried out for the school team and I believed I had played exceptionally well and would undoubtedly make the roster. The names of those who made the team were posted next to the coach's office. Not seeing my name on that list was devastating. A few weeks later a team member got injured and I was asked to fill in for him. My stubborn streak surfaced and I told the coach to go to hell. I was too proud to accept his offer, probably not the best decision as I loved hockey.

During my final year of high school I learned how to drive and booked an appointment with the police department for a driving test. The parking aspect of the test went fine. Now for the road test. As I drove down the street the officer told me to turn left. I did so while a car approached a good distance away in the opposite direction. Immediately I was commanded to return to the police station because I should have waited for the car to pass before turning left. I was seventeen and stubborn. Close to the station I deliberately drove over a curb. "Now," I said glaring at the officer. "You have a reason to fail me."

Twice more I took the driver's test with the same police officer with no chance of passing. The fourth try was successful as another officer tested me. Sometimes it pays to keep your mouth shut.

During high school I was thinking that I would go to university and study to become a lawyer. I had always enjoyed helping people and I had had a few run-ins with the police so I thought why not try this as a career. I also thought about just travelling after high school. I tried to talk my buddies into buying an old aluminum bread truck and just jump in it and see where it would take us. I couldn't get anyone to go along with me. Many other career paths entered my head, they left my mind nearly as soon as they entered it but being a lawyer was one that would continue to cross my mind.

I completed high school at the age of seventeen with an eighty percent average, applied for and was accepted to university for that Fall. That summer before university my cousin and I visited our uncle in Toronto. The two-week vacation turned into three months. We indulged in all the activities you're not supposed to at our age. We did drugs, booze and partied all night. The days we weren't partying I would often jump on the subway and get off at different locations of the city. I wanted to experience different cultures and this was a way to do that. I enjoyed these excursions around the city. I met many people and never once did I run into trouble. People for the most part were friendly and only too glad to have a conversation. The end of the summer lurked around the corner, and I played with the idea of remaining in Toronto. My mother would call and inquire when I was coming home as university was starting soon. I'd often listen to Rod Stewart's song "Maggie May" and wonder what I should do in my circumstance. The song is about a young man who has a decision to make about school. The party life was ever enticing. I was seventeen and having the time of my life. Once again, as in Grade one, school would get in the way of having fun.

I told my mother I was thinking about staying permanently in Toronto. One week later she arrives at my uncle's doorstep. That same day my uncle and I went for a drive. We each smoked a joint and he was so stoned he drove the wrong way on a divided highway. We laughed so much our eyes watered. I was stoned and I really didn't see the danger of our situation. Once back at my uncle's place my mother could tell something was wrong. I guess mother's instinct rose to the surface and she said: "That's it. You're going home." I believed she literally saved my life that day. If I had stayed in Toronto doing drugs and drinking, I firmly believe it would have eventually killed me. I'm not sure what the guy in Rod Stewart's song did but I know through my mother's intervention I made the best decision. One that would change my life.

So, home I went in early September 1974. I reconnected with the friends I had in high school. I started university still with the thought of becoming a lawyer. The first year in university went well and I partied like all students do.

One weekend I was out with my friends having a great time. On the way back home from the party I fell asleep in the back seat. I was awoken by loud noises and people screaming. I looked out the car window and my friends were involved in a fight. My friends later told me the guys they were fighting had tried to run them of the road. I jumped out of the car to help but as I did some girl hit me in the face with a bottle. Blood ran down my face and I couldn't see anything. When my eyes cleared my friends were gone and I was alone. The group my friends were fighting spotted me and began to attack me. I was alone and there wasn't much I could do. Later on my friends returned and found me on the ground behind their car. I woke up in hospital with a broken jaw, a broken nose and broken ribs. I had surgery the next day to repair my broken jaw. My father showed up at the ER but I couldn't tell him the truth of what happened. The next day I was released.

I was angry at my friends for leaving me behind that night. For weeks I refused to talk to them. They were good friends but I couldn't get over the fact they had left me there all alone. Once again my father came to the rescue. My father never talked about his time in the war. He never participated in military parades; he never requested his military medals from WWII. My brother, Michael (Mick) would request them after our father's death. To our surprise there were five medals each representing major battles he had faught in during the war.

My father had observed my disappointment in my friends, and one day he told me he had a story he wanted me to hear. I just want you to listen my father said, no questions. I agreed. He went on to tell me about friends of his in the war. Many of them were young kids just like he was. When in battle some of them would freeze up and just lie down on the ground and refuse to fight. Some of them would lose control of their bodily functions. My father told me he forgave them, he said sometimes fear takes over and you do things you're not proud of. I had so many questions for him. This was the first time my father had ever talked about the war. I couldn't ask him any as I had promised I wouldn't. He walked away and left me with that story. I contemplated what he had told me and the next day I phoned my friends. We are still friends to this day.

I had completed one year of university when my buddy from Grade nine, the one who I had helped with Math was back home. We reconnected and became friends once again. During my second year of university he introduced me to Darlene, who would later become my wife. Sometimes things happen for a good reason. Sometimes kindness finds its way back to you. My friend would eventually move away and we haven't seen each other in over forty years. I'm not sure if he is even still alive. I hope he is and that he is doing well.

After my second year of university I took the semester off. My father said computers were the way of the future and he suggested I do a computer course. He said I just couldn't sit around the house and do nothing with my life. I registered for a two year computer studies course at the local community college. I completed the course and found employment with a local technology company. A few months later I realized this type of work wasn't for me. I quit that job and returned to university.

Darlene and I continued dating and our relationship was beginning to get serious. In the early years we just had fun and enjoyed life. We partied with our friends. We spent many weekends camping in the local parks. We went to all the local dances and all our friends and families weddings. I would occasionally go drinking with my buddies and forget to pick her up for our date. She would always forgive me. I'm sure there were many times she wanted to just walk away from our relationship but was I ever lucky she didn't.

She stayed in there and I am the person I am today because of her. Many relationships fall apart but sometimes you have to work at it in order to keep it together. We were three years into our relationship and she had begun to give me the purpose in life I had been searching for. She grounded me, she made me happy and we were great together. My second shot at university went great. During my last term at university we decided to get married. I studied for my final exams and Darlene planned our wedding. I finished my exams on April 23rd, 1982 and we got married May 8th 1982. I graduated with a degree in Economics with a Business Minor. Sad that I hadn't become a lawyer but happy I had my degree and I was married to a beautiful, wonderful woman.

We had a free bar at our wedding which of course was a crowd pleaser. For obvious reasons I abstained from alcohol consumption at the wedding. The next night we hosted a party at our apartment, and I made up for the lack of alcohol the night before. The flight to Florida the next morning was no picnic for my wife, as this was her first time on a plane. Unfortunately, I was too sick (actually hung over is more accurate) to help calm her fear of flying. To make matters worse, arriving in Florida, the rental car had no air conditioning. So here we were, I was hung over. It was hotter than I had ever experienced, and we were lost. We should have asked for a map. The situation struck both of us as hilarious. We looked at each other and laughed. We were in Florida on our honeymoon. Who cared about little disruptions? Eventually, we found our way to the beach and to our hotel. I thought to myself how did we manage to pay for the wedding and the honeymoon? I just finished university and didn't have a job. We just got married and now here we are in Florida. For some reason, even to this day, we have always managed to enjoy our lives not worrying too much about money. Things always seemed to work out for us.

On the second day in Florida my wife waited in the car while I went into a Burger King for the first time. At that time we didn't have a Burger King back home. I read out loud the items on the menu as I was deciding which to choose. Next thing I see the waitress handing me two large bags full of hamburgers and french fries. Unknown to me she was cashing in every food item I'd read out loud. Too embarrassed to explain the situation I took the bags and paid the exorbitant bill. My wife laughed so hard she almost choked on a french fry. We ate hamburgers and fries every day for the next week. We still laugh about that to this day.

Darlene was employed at an Insurance company, however, six months into our marriage I hadn't been able to secure employment. We made the tough decision to move to Toronto. I was about to drive to the airport to book the tickets when I received a letter from the Federal government inviting me to an interview for a job, I had the interview and was offered the job. I began work in January 1983. I often wonder how our lives would have turned out had I not received that letter that day. I worked for the Federal government for thirty years before retiring at the age of fifty-six.

Life was good. We travelled every year and were delighted when our two sons were born, Bobby in October 1985 and Josh in April 1993. Nothing is ever perfect, though. In between the boys my wife lost our baby girl when she was eight months pregnant. That August day in 1990 shook our world. We went from planning our baby's birth to losing her. The day we lost our baby girl my wife was placed on a maternity ward. We could hear mothers in their rooms, their baby's crying. We decided at that moment to leave the hospital. My wife got dressed and we walked out of the hospital. For two years my wife talked very little about what had happened until one day she started to shake. I took her to the hospital and we realized that the trauma of losing our child had caught up with her. We returned home and I immediately booked a trip to Florida. We decided to try again for a baby and nine months later in April, 1993 our son Josh was born healthy. Those nine months were the longest of our lives. We constantly worried if something would happen again. The loss and the heartache have never completely gone away. It's been over thirty years and we both still grieve the loss. I wonder if our baby girl had lived would we have had our younger son Josh. I would like to think the answer would be yes.

I'm not a religious person, however every night I prayed for good health for my wife, my mother and siblings and my wife's family. When my sons came along, I added them to the list. My priorities shifted as I prayed that if my family was destined to be burdened with a serious illness that it would be me. I'd had a fulfilling life and wanted my children to be given the same gift. I wanted my wife to be there for them, sons need their mother. Little did I know that prayer would be answered.

Darlene and I built our cabin and bought our home. We went on many vacations often accompanied by my mother who really enjoyed going on trips with us. In general, life was good.

We had the normal life worries, such as how the children were doing in school. Could we afford to enroll them in their favorite sport? Could we afford university when the time came? Do they have good, reliable friends? Were they getting into trouble? Doing drugs?

I never worried about my health and when I turned forty I started jogging. I would run the five miles home from work every day. I lost forty pounds and felt great as it gave me a sense of peace that I was doing the right thing to maintain a healthy life. I understood the older one gets the more careful one has to be about health issues, especially when you have your wife and children depending on you. I will admit jogging was hard at first as my body ached all over and I would come up with any excuse to quit. The rain, wind, cold and the snow were top of the list of excuses. My wife encouraged me to continue to run. Eventually I reached a point where a snowstorm wouldn't prevent me from the enjoyment of jogging. Running would give me a natural high. I would continue jogging for the next ten years.

I truly believe those early life experiences helped me become the person I am today. I was a stubborn, fearless child. I grew into a young boy who feared nothing and loved life and having fun. I brought that same fearlessness, stubbornness and love of life into my adult years. That stubbornness, love of life and the love of my wife and sons gave me the will and strength to fight for my life. Remember your life, your childhood, how you loved life and having fun, and draw on those experiences in your fight to survive.

2

THE CANCER DIAGNOSIS

I n 2006 I'm fifty years old, still running and in the best shape of my life. I rarely have reason to see our family doctor. My son Joshua (thirteen years old at the time) had a sore throat so I brought him to see the doctor. As usual, Josh was diagnosed with strep throat, a recurring illness he suffered from since childhood. While there I asked the doctor to check me out as well. He asked the usual questions then checked my heart and blood pressure, and referred me for blood work. A week later I returned confident all was well for I was rarely sick.

I sat across from the doctor's desk as he read out the individual tests saying that each was normal. He suddenly paused and looked at me, a look I'd never seen before and for the first time in my life I was worried about my health. He looked back to the results and read out the level of my Prostate Specific Antigen (PSA) test which was 6.8. A normal range for my age group is approximately 2.5. He then performed a rectum digital exam. I was relieved when he said the prostrate didn't feel enlarged. However, he said that as he was a general practitioner, I should seek the advice of a specialist.

He booked an appointment for me to see an urologist. The two-week waiting period was grueling as I felt vulnerable and scared that perhaps for the first time in my life, I could be faced with a serious health problem. My sense of feeling invincible had finally run out. The urologist performed a digital exam as well and commented that the prostate did feel normal. He suggested my raised PSA could be due to an infection and prescribed antibiotics for a two-week period. Another blood test was ordered to check my PSA. There was very little change, and the urologist prescribed a second round of antibiotics. He explained sometimes it takes several doses to clear up an infection. My PSA level was still elevated and a third round of antibiotics was prescribed.

This course of treatment lasted six months. By this time, I'd become frustrated and rather concerned that something more serious was wrong. On my next visit the urologist once again recommended antibiotics. I refused and asked to have a biopsy. He agreed and two weeks later I had the biopsy completed. Three weeks later I'm called into his office with the final diagnosis. I had prostate cancer. After a brief discussion of options he recommended removal of the prostate. My wife and I agreed. I'm fifty years old and more terrified than I've ever been in my life. My mother's brother had died from prostate cancer at fifty-two years old.

There are side effects men face once the prostate is removed. The most profound is that nerves can be severed rendering intercourse impossible. This could mean the end of an intimate relationship with my wife. We've always shared a healthy sex life and this possibility was a major concern. My wife was forty-six at the time and looked great.

I discussed this possibility with her, and she responded with these exact words: "Bob, if the nerves are severed, we will work things out. There are always other options, other ways to enjoy each other intimately. I would rather have you alive."

My surgery was successful with no lasting side effects. The surgeon explained how truly lucky I was as the cancer in the prostate was identified as "voluptuous," meaning it had consumed the whole prostate yet the cancer hadn't spread outside the prostate. I didn't need radiation or chemotherapy. He stated I was lucky to have my prostate checked when I did. Without question, my son's strep throat saved my life. I didn't have symptoms, and by the time they appeared chances are it would have been too late to save me. My son Josh saved my life that day. Josh would turn out to be my savior on a number of occasions. Early detection is crucial. Men should have their PSA checked by at least 50 years old. Sooner if you have an increased family risk of Prostate Cancer.

For the next six years I underwent numerous blood tests to check my PSA levels at three-month, six-month and once a year intervals. The stress and anxiety waiting for those results became unbearable. The once care-free man who never worried about his health became someone who obsessed over it. My wife's love, support and understanding got me through those years, literally preventing me from losing my mind. Four years later in 2010 I finally begin to feel like my old self and I resumed jogging. My PSA blood tests are now done once a year. The stress of waiting for tests results was always brutal. I finally have come to terms with the fact that worry will change nothing, though this old adage is true: It's easier said than done. I'm still not sure if time has made me less of a worrier. I try to live as normal a life as possible while fighting off the fear that if my PSA level soars this could indicate that the cancer has spread to other organs. During those years my wife was supportive and understanding. She stood by me and was patient. The intimacy between us returned and exists to this day.

The summer of 2010 I accompanied my oldest son Bobby to a motorcycle shop. He intended to purchase a Crotch Rocket motorcycle. I always wanted a motorcycle myself and while there, I saw one I instantly fell in love with. Without consulting my wife, I bought the bike. Darlene was, shall we say, somewhat displeased. She understood this lifelong desire and made me promise that if I had an accident and survived, I would end my motorcycle riding days. I reluctantly agreed, completed the motorcycle safety course, and passed the road test on the first attempt. Being older and wiser I don't make unwanted comments to the tester as I did during my driver's license test. For two years I enjoyed the daily excursions on my bike. Darlene only occasionally rode with me as she complained the seat was way too uncomfortable.

One sunny summer afternoon in 2012 I'm riding along on my Yamaha V-Star 1100 bike in an easterly direction towards downtown when a woman in a huge Chevrolet Yukon runs a stop sign and pulls out onto the main road in front of me. I'm travelling at fifty kilometers an hour. I'm wearing a white t-shirt and jeans. I also have on my helmet and leather gloves.

I'm heading straight for the Yukon. I have no time to react. What do I do? My brain is flooded with options. Sudden braking will cause me to T-bone the truck. I'll hit the curve if I turn to the right. Neither option was a viable one. I pull to the right, put the bike down on its side and slide about thirty feet with the bike on top of me. My right leg, hip, arm, and shoulder receive burns from the pavement. I'm sliding towards a utility pole, about to crash into it. Is this how I die? To this day I don't know why or how I missed the pole. Neither am I sure how the Chevrolet Yukon didn't hit me. The woman later said she hadn't seen me or the bike.

The police, ambulance and fire truck arrive. Besides the scrapes and burns on my right side my left thumb is also broken. The police officer tells me I'm lucky not to have T-boned the truck as I most likely would have broken my neck and legs. Strangely a week later a young kid T-boned a truck on his motorcycle and died. I survived a tragedy once again not really knowing the reason why.

I miss my motorcycle and the "one note sound of the engine." This expression was a joke between me and Darlene. We argued every time Bob Seager's song "Turn the Page" came on the radio. I would say the song was about a guy on a motorcycle traveling the country and she would say it was about a band in a bus touring the country playing different concerts. Every time she was on the bike I would say "Can't you hear the one note sound of the engine." She'd laugh and roll her eyes. I miss the drives around the city and along the countryside with the ocean on one side. As I rode my bike alone most times, I called myself a member of the Lonesome Riders Club. Every time my wife and I would see someone riding their motorcycle alone I would joke that they were a member of my Lonesome Riders Club. As much as I loved the motorcycle, I had to keep the promise I made to my wife. That was one promise I hated to keep but I did.

Shortly after the motorcycle accident I began to experience dizzy spells and disorientation. I put these symptoms down to the after effects of the accident. The feelings persist but I am determined to stay positive nevertheless.

In the fall of 2012 I find out the Eagles are scheduled to perform in Las Vegas in November at the MGM Grand Hotel. I've been a huge fan of the band since high school. I'm fifty-six and have never seen them live in concert. I discuss with Darlene about going to Vegas and she is as excited as me. What a lifetime experience that will be! We buy VIP concert tickets which cost a fortune. I want to sit close enough to the stage that if Joe Walsh, one of the best guitarists in the world, drops his guitar pick I can actually see it fall.

We arrived in Vegas in November of 2012 and have reservations for the "Paris" hotel which is located on the famous Vegas Strip. As this is our first trip to Vegas we are amazed at the sites and atmosphere of the city. People laughing, excited and having fun. We walk along the Strip the first night. Women are passing out cards and I take them not knowing what they were for. I soon realize what they are advertising. Anyone who's ever visited Vegas will understand what I mean. I'm very happy with my wife so no need to use any of the cards.

We do the normal things visitors do in Vegas: Gamble in the casinos, see the shows, and dine out. Life is wonderful. I learned how to play blackjack, and by the time the vacation neared its end, I was betting one hundred and eighty dollars a hand. I won enough money to pay for the Eagles tickets. We celebrated Darlene's birthday (November 18th) by ordering room service and making love.

The day of the Eagles concert arrives, and I spend the day singing all their songs in anticipation. I'm as excited like I was seventeen again. We are in the front row and Glenn Frey, Don Henley and the rest of the band walk out onto the stage. All the difficult times of my life fade away. The prostate cancer, the motorcycle accident, losing our baby and even the dizziness are forgotten. I feel young again and I'm living my dream with my wife, my best friend by my side. I couldn't imagine anywhere else I would rather be, although maybe sitting in the back room having a beer with the Eagles would have been pretty good.

The Eagles perform all their hit songs to a packed MGM theatre. We laughed and sang along. Don Henley ended the show with the song "Desperado." I cried tears of joy that night, beyond thrilled to be at an Eagles concert. If that had been the only thing we did in Vegas, the trip would have been well worth the expense.

The next day we drove to the Grand Canyon and stopped off at the Hoover Dam. The only word I can use to appropriately express these two sites is stunning. As with all good things the vacation ended. There are several details of the trip I have omitted. For as the saying goes "What happens in Vegas stays in Vegas!"

As soon as we return home my dizziness, disorientation, and worry kicks in, which becomes a routine part of my existence. The yearly blood tests for my PSA level continues. The results are normal, therefore as dumb as it may sound; I assumed my symptoms weren't serious. If the prostate cancer had spread to other organs, it would have shown up in the blood tests. As I reflect on that time, it was foolish and stupid not to tell the doctor about how I was feeling. I returned to work and my co-workers noticed I was not myself. They said I looked worried all the time. I confided in them how I felt and one lady I was close to gave me a religious medal with the word hope on one side and the picture of an angel on the other. Our cottage neighbour in the country heard my story about the medal and she gave me one as well with an angel and a red heart. My mother also presented me with a medallion of a baby angel. I'm not religious, yet somehow, the medals gave me hope, hope they would bring me good luck. I carried them to every blood test.

I confided to my son Josh that I feared losing the medals and he suggested to have their image tattooed on my arm. It was a great idea and I had them tattooed on my left shoulder along with the names of both sons and my wife. I added a cloud with rays of sunlight shining through to represent my sister Joan who passed away in 2008. This cloud and rays of sunshine later brought me peace, reminding me of loved ones who'd passed away: my parents, my sister Joan, my brother Wayne and my best friend Mike. Hopefully they were all in heaven and looking out for all those they left behind.

I retired from work in February of 2013. In July there was an outdoor music concert within driving distance from where we lived. As fate would have it the Eagles headlined the event. Of course, Darlene and I booked our VIP tickets and drove the hundred or so miles to the event. The day was extremely hot with a packed venue. The Eagles played for two hours. I was bothered that their onstage presence was quite different from the time in Vegas. It wasn't overly obvious, but being an avid fan I noticed they didn't interact in their usual friendly manner. My son Josh said perhaps spending so much time together eventually leads to animosity. Perhaps they now performed together for the sake of the music and the money. Sadly, I agreed.

On December 19, 2013 everything changed for me. It had been a little over six years since conquering prostate cancer. The day began as normal with the persistent dizziness and strange sensations I'd experienced for the past two years. I visited my sister that morning and returned home for lunch. A short while later I was suddenly struck by a terrible pain in my lower right side. The pain worsened until it became excruciating. Josh, who was twenty at the time, tried to help me, but I snapped at him to leave me alone. I lay down on my bed. The pain grew more unbearable, and I began to shake uncontrollably. Josh persisted in his attempt to help me and once again I shouted at him to leave me alone. God bless him he didn't listen and he called his mother at work. If he hadn't made that call, I most likely would have died. My wife was at a Christmas lunch with her co-workers. She left and came straight home and phoned our oldest son Bobby. I was in racks of pain and didn't want to move. I was prepared to die, if need be, to escape the awful pain and discomfort. Bobby was twenty–six at the time. He, along with Josh and Darlene ignored my protests and lifted me from the bed.

My mother who lived with us for over twenty seven years often looked out the window of her apartment. In order to prevent her from seeing my condition my family sneaked me out to the car. Darlene didn't call an ambulance sensing I needed to reach the hospital sooner rather than later. That decision saved my life.

The emergency room was full. I sat in a wheelchair doubled over with pain unable to look up at the nurse to answer her questions. She realized I was in distress and wheeled me inside where the doctor immediately saw me. He suspected I had a ruptured appendix. I was relieved as I thought it was something more serious, however the pain and discomfort intensified. The nurse gave me a morphine shot which eased the pain somewhat. I was sent for a CT Scan. My wife waited in an inside room of the ER. My sons weren't allowed in so they went home at their mother's insistence.

I was chatting with Darlene when the curtain around

the bed opened to reveal a male and female doctor. They had the results of the CT scan. I held Darlene's hand thinking I needed surgery for a ruptured appendix. What they would say is still etched in my memory like an engraving on a headstone. I still wake up at night and relive that scene, the words they say echoing in my head. "Mr. Abbott, we have the results of your CT scan. It's not good news. You will have a hard fight ahead of you. The results show you have colon cancer, and it looks like it has metastasized to your liver and lungs. The blood work and CT scan shows your bowel has ruptured and you are septic. You were lucky to get here when you did. If you had waited another hour, you would have died."

The doctors then simply turned without uttering another word and left. Darlene and I hold hands, we stare at each other in complete shock and disbelief. We both cry. I looked into her eyes and said: "There go our dreams, our life plans, our travel plans, seeing Josh graduate university, seeing our boys marry, holding our grandchildren." Devastation doesn't capture how we felt at that moment. There are no words to describe the feeling that engulfs you when you're told you have cancer that has spread and the outlook for survival isn't looking good. You're consumed with panic, fear, emptiness, and shock. The feeling that you're outside your body. It's both overwhelming and frightening how your life can change in a matter of moments. You wonder if this is real. Am I dreaming? How did this happen to me? You search for answers but there are none. I could hardly speak and when I did, I didn't recognize my own voice. I thought how do I break this devastating news to my sons, my mother, and my brothers, and sisters. It was 1:00 am and we had to let people know what was happening. Darlene called my brother, Mick and asked him to come to the hospital.

Within a short time Mick arrives with his wife, Sandy. We tell them the devastating news and my dire prognosis. They are in utter disbelief and struggle to find the right words. I ask them would they break the news to our mother and the rest of the family, they agree. We will talk to our sons, Bobby and Josh.

After Mick and Sandy left I was floundering with nowhere to hide. I couldn't run. I couldn't close my eyes and believe this death sentence wasn't real. My life had been in an instant turned inside out and I didn't know what to do or how to react. You hear these stories of death but you never believe you will become the main character in the story. It's always about someone else not you. This time it was about me and I was completely devastated.

I'd known Darlene for thirty-six years. I'd seen her cry twice, when we lost our baby girl and when her mother died. Now tears flowed down her face. Suddenly it struck me in this terrible moment, something positive had happened. It was the fact that I loved my wife even more if that was possible and I realized she truly loved me. All I could think about was how much I would miss her. Miss our chats at night in bed watching a movie. Miss our conversation on our Sunday drives. Miss our walks in the park. Miss our vacations together. Miss the Florida sunsets. We were always close, but I believe that crushing news brought us even closer.

A short while later I was brought up to a private room and scheduled for emergency surgery to remove the cancer in my bowel. Due to septicemia (infection in the blood) the surgery was delayed for a day and a half. I was injected with antibiotics and given several blood transfusions in an effort to raise my hemoglobin and potassium to the point where I'd have a fighting chance to survive the surgery. The delay in surgery proved to be beneficial as the doctor who was scheduled to perform my surgery was called away to another emergency. A younger doctor was called in to replace him. For reasons I can't really explain I had more confidence in the younger surgeon.

During the delay, blood work was taken at various intervals to see if the antibiotics were clearing up the septicemia. One minute the results were good, the next time not so good and the surgery was cancelled yet again. There was no way I'd survive surgery with bacteria flowing through my blood. Based on my conversations with the doctor, my chances of surviving surgery were extremely low.

I felt it was time to say a final good-bye to Darlene, my sons Bobby and Josh, my brothers and sisters, and my eighty-two-year-old mother who'd already lost a daughter.

I discussed my life insurances and outstanding bills, reassuring Darlene the money from these insurances after my death would pay off all our debts. I felt the need to warn her about taking precautions if she met another man, to be careful about their intentions, particularly in money matters. She was fifty-three and looked thirty. My siblings often joked they couldn't understand how I snagged such a pretty woman.

It may sound selfish but the thought of another man lounging on the deck of our cabin with a beer in his hand watching the setting sun over the pond with Darlene beside him bothered me. I had built that cabin piece by piece with just a hammer and a hand saw like Johnny Cash, the country music singer says in his song "One Piece at a Time." Many weekends friends would help, and in truth, it's thanks to them the cabin was finally completed. My main goal was to ensure it went to my sons. Darlene promised it would stay in the family. She said she'd never be with another man, but

I realized time does eventually lessen grief. I'd spent the better part of our marriage of my life doing my best to make her happy. All I asked was that she visit my grave once in a while and keep it maintained.

I then spoke to my sons asking them to take care of their mother, yet at the same time do their best to fulfill their own dreams and aspirations. Bobby was working and doing well while Josh was attending university. I expressed my love for them and told them that life must go on, and to enjoy theirs as much as possible. I told my mother how much I loved her and how I wanted her not to grieve to the point it affected her health. I also asked her to make sure Darlene was okay. My siblings along with several of their children came to my room and we spoke about what was happening to me. I said I loved them and asked them to keep an eye on Darlene and my sons.

From 1:30 pm on Thursday December 19th to 9:00 pm Friday December 20th, 2013, my life had done a complete turnabout. I went from living to preparing for a surgery I would most likely not survive. I went from having dreams with my family to saying a possible last good-bye to them. It was the hardest thing I have or would ever experience in my life.

Fortunately, my septicemia cleared up and at 9:00 pm I was brought down to the operating room for surgery. My entire family watched the nurses roll me towards the eleva-tor. I thought this maybe the last time I see them. Doubtless they thought the same. As the elevator doors were closing Darlene made eye contact with me and I saw love, fear and loneliness in them. I felt so alone, so helpless, the urge to cry overwhelmed me. I wanted to jump off the stretcher and run, unable to believe what was happening.

I prayed to my deceased sister, Joan and to my father,

Ron. If you're in heaven, please know I need your help. At such a critical moment in life you reach out to whatever or whomever can help. You try to cling to life, to grasp for that little bit of hope that while you're alive you still have a chance.

Suddenly, I'm in the operating room and being moved onto the table. The young surgeon smiles and says, "It's about time you're here. I've been waiting all day." His smile and casual comment helped me relax, that I was in good hands. Before he began the surgery, he explained the three possible outcomes. 1) I could die during surgery. 2) I could survive with a bag on my side. 3) The surgery would be a complete success with most of my bowel intact. Regardless I would still have to deal with my liver and lung cancer. My only statement to him was "Do your best."

My family, siblings and their spouses sat in a room waiting for the surgery to end. My wife told me several hours had passed when a nurse came to the waiting room. Everyone thought she would tell us the outcome of the surgery. To their dismay it hadn't even begun. A specialist had been called in as an unexpected issue had come up, the nurse didn't specify. Fearful that this wasn't a good sign everyone remained until 2:00 am to hear the outcome of the surgery.

Over five hours later in the early hours of December 21st, hooked up to all sorts of tubes and wires I was brought to the Special Care Unit. Darlene later told me she'd been overcome by how sick and pale I looked and truly thought I would never wake up. I finally awoke with a nurse sitting next to my bed, assigned to maintain a constant watch over me. Darlene and our boys stood next to me. I was alive. I had survived. I was surprised I was still alive but the reality of what was ahead of me scared me beyond description. I moved my hand to see if I had a bag on my side. Darlene noticed this and assured me I didn't. We all cried with happiness. I had fought one battle and won; yet had a more frightening journey ahead of me. At least I had a chance to fight. At least that's what I thought.

3

CAN I SLOW DOWN TIME?

Darlene stayed by my side morning and night for three days waiting to see if I would live. Exhausted and relieved I had survived she finally went home to rest. Later, on December 21st, 2013, I was moved to a semi-private room. As Christmas was only a few days away, most patients had been released and I had the room to myself. Alone for the first time since surgery, my mind was flooded with all sorts of thoughts. I'd beaten the odds and survived the surgery. Even though I was nauseated and in pain, I thought perhaps there was a chance this cancer would not kill me.

At that very moment the doctor who first saw me in the Emergency Room walks in. I can still recall the events of that day. I'm lying there with tubes running from my nose and mouth. I'm hooked up to an intravenous line. I've just gotten through surgery that I wasn't supposed to survive. Without even a hello or how are you feeling he proceeds to explain my condition. There's no sign of compassion or feeling on his face or in his voice. He says the colon surgery was successful; however there are five spots on the right side of my liver each measuring five centimeters. There are also five spots on my right lung and two on my left lung. He goes on to say that my chance of survival is slim. I will have a hard fight ahead of me. He then walks away leaving me alone to ponder what he has just told me. Basically he has just given me a death sentence.

I fall back into the pillows. I am weak, desperate, and alone. I couldn't speak, my voice had deserted me. This doctor had ripped away my hope of living. I reflect on my life. For some unexplainable reason the good times are forgotten and the bad memories resurface. I have survived three car accidents. I survived the crazy life I lived in Toronto. I survived a brutal police beating. I survived prostate cancer. I survived a motorcycle accident. I'm not sure why I survived all this, now cancer is coming for me once again. This is not the news I wanted to hear especially after the last few days which I've spent struggling to hold on to life. My hope has been crushed by a doctor who laid out my bleak future in a monotone, uncaring voice. Maybe I'm being too unkind. Maybe that was his way of coping with news he most likely has to deliver on a daily or weekly basis. Or maybe that's who he is.

Christmas is four days away and here I am in hospital trying to recover, thinking this will most likely be my last one. I try to force myself to believe that I'm not going home for one last Christmas. How do you summon up the hope, the strength to partake in festive activities in such circumstances?

Darlene arrives back at the hospital, and I give her the news. With her help and support we agree to put all my energy into recovering from the bowel surgery and make a real effort to enjoy Christmas. I'll hold off until the new year to even consider beginning the "hard fight ahead of me."

I'm anxious to go home and ask the nurse what I can do to speed up my recovery and leave the hospital. She says to get out of bed as soon as possible and get active. For the next five days I walked at least twenty miles up and down the corridor. Two o'clock in the morning the nurses at the station would smile and say, "There he goes again." I walked so much my doctor advised me to get more rest. No, I tell myself. Walking is a way of getting me home faster, so no way was I going to ease up.

Friends and family visited often during those hospital days. All were polite and tried to talk about ordinary things, yet I saw the worry and sorrow in their eyes they couldn't hide. The worry and sorrow that I was going to die. Darlene remained each day until midnight. We'd talk about the past, about paying off bills if I didn't make it. We watched movies on her laptop. We talked about making sure Bobby and Josh would be okay. All we wanted was for them to be happy. I wanted Darlene to assure me she would leave the cabin to our sons. I knew Darlene would be okay, she was and still is the strongest person I know.

Darlene's positive attitude and our son's determination to keep me alive helped me through that first week and everything that would follow. I owe my life to my wife and sons and to the great doctor who performed the colon surgery. He later confided to me that he'd only had two inches of bowel to reattach to the section from which he'd removed the cancer. What if the much older, original surgeon had performed the operation? Would he have felt that two inches was enough for the reattachment? Would I have ended up with a permanent bag on my side? Would I have died during surgery?

I spent Christmas day in hospital. Darlene wanted to bring in my gifts and put up a little tree. I adamantly refused and say I want to open them at home in a warm, familiar place with my family. Not where I felt close to death. Finally, on Boxing Day, after spending seven days in hospital I'm free to go home. Before I go home the surgeon gives me a follow-up appointment to see him on January 6, 2014, to learn the results of the bowel tissue samples he sent to the laboratory. Darlene and Josh pick me up from the hospital. I'm experiencing so many emotions at this time that I can't really explain any one in particular.

When I open the door to our house, Tigi, our Pitbull, is standing at the top of the stairs. Her reaction when she sees me is completely amazing. As I walked up the steps she ran back and forth in front of me with her tail wagging so fast it was almost a blur. When I sat in the living room chair, she jumped up on my lap. She'd never done that before. Whenever I moved to another part of the house, she would follow me. Each time I went to the bathroom, she'd wait outside the door. I was amazed and touched by her attention and concern for me. It was as if she knew I wasn't well and wanted to protect me. To be honest, I was never much of an animal person. Tigi changed all that for me. Actually, as I write this story, she's lying on the floor beside me. She's now fifteen years old. They say a dog lives longer when it is loved. Tigi has many years left in her yet.

Now that I'm home I open my Christmas gifts, thinking again this will most likely be my last. At this precise moment sudden fear and panic grips me. It's difficult to try and recover from surgery with the idea that death is close at hand. This constant fear of death never leaves my mind.

Taking a shower is a challenge, it exhausts me and I'm forced to lie down. I can't believe what's become of my life. I've gone from being in good physical condition to being wiped out following a shower. I'm resting in bed thinking all this when Tigi jumps onto the bed and lies next to me. For a brief moment her presence wipes away those desperate feelings.

For the next few weeks, I manage to get through the day without dwelling too much on my situation. The nights close in and I'm alone with my frightening thoughts. Even as I try, I can't adequately describe the level of anxiety, fear and panic that consumes me, overpowers me. I shudder at all I'll miss. Future travels, our sons' weddings, their children being born. I'm heart sick at the idea all this will occur without me. I think, could I have done more with my sons? I remember Bobby's baseball games and Josh's hockey games. The years taking both of them to swimming lessons. I think about our family vacations. I think did I do enough with them? Was I a good father? I hoped I was.

Darlene and I had had a happy, productive life up to this point. Now I was searching for something, anything. Was it hope? Was it God? I'd had the images from the religious medals tattooed on my shoulder, yet that wasn't enough. Our cabin neighbor who lived close to us in the city was a deeply religious woman and was known to bless sick people who had run out of options. She offered to give me her blessing. As I've stated I'm not overly religious, but I was searching for anything to give me hope, something to cling to.

Darlene and I went to her home. She took me aside and proceeded to bless me. To my astonishment I experienced a profound sense of peace, and a chill passed through my entire body. Perhaps I thought afterwards it was merely me grasping for something to hold onto. Though, as I write about this, I'm more than ever convinced I did experience something. Something that I'm at a loss to explain.

Time is drawing close for the meeting with the doctor

which will determine whether I'll live or die, you want time to slow down. The thought of that meeting scares me beyond description. The nights are the most difficult because it means that another day has come and gone. My life may soon be over. Everything seems to happen in an instant. I panic because the days speed by. This is the one aspect of my illness Darlene could not understand. I felt as each day passed I was getting closer to death. You take time for granted not thinking each second, each minute, each hour, each day could be your last. That thought scares me and hardly ever leaves my mind, even ten years later. My drives with Darlene were a way I could slow down time. You don't see the passage of time in the trees, in the birds flying overhead, in the water lapping to the shore on a quiet pond. No matter how many drives we go on, the day we dread the most, January 6th, is upon us. I thought nothing could get worse. But it did.

Darlene and I sit in the waiting room to see the surgeon who now had the results of the biopsy of my tissue samples. The surgeon's intern came in and told us the cancer was confined to the colon and hadn't spread. We were ecstatic. I was out of danger. I was going to live a long life. In that instant we began to think about our dreams once again. I thought I had my life back again. We were very happy to hear this news because it wasn't what we had expected. All the worry was for nothing. In less than two minutes we would once again be blindsided, devastated. The intern left and the surgeon came in. He asked if the intern had given us the results. He paused and stared at us. I guess he could tell by our look of relief and happiness there had been some kind of miscommunication.

He gave us the true results. The bowel cancer had metastasized to my liver and both lungs. It was quite obvious by his expression he felt terrible for the mistake and profusely apologized. To this day I have no idea why the intern said what he said. Neither did I press the issue. The surgeon referred me to an oncologist and said he'd keep himself informed about my file to ensure the cancer clinic took good care of me. He reiterated that my chance for survival was slim to none. I asked if this new cancer was related to my prostate cancer to which he replied it was a completely separate issue. I left the surgeon's office with an appointment to see the oncologist mid-February 2014.

Darlene and I left heart sick, literally physically weakened. Imagine one minute being told you're cured then the next minute told that it was a mistake. The bleak reality is that I'd been handed a death sentence again. It was official. I couldn't deny my fate anymore. I was going to die. I felt like I floated outside my body. Everything was surreal. I had to make plans for my death. I could only guess how Darlene felt. Her husband, her life partner of thirty-seven years, her best friend, her lover, the father of her children would soon be snatched away. Her dreams were my dreams. All that was going to end. I was scared, desperate. Once again I wanted to run, to hide. You go from being given your life back to it being snatched away again in two minutes. I walked out of the hospital speechless. I tried to speak to Darlene but the words wouldn't come out. When they did it sounded like a different person. As I walked from the hospital to our car I felt like I wasn't there. I felt like I was above the clouds looking down. It felt like I had already died.

When we get home we give our sons the bad news. It was like they've been hit by a two-ton truck. They didn't know what to say. It was devastating. It was the hardest thing that we ever had to tell them. I have a CT scan done in early February and wait for the results. Perhaps when I speak to the oncologist to discuss the CT scan she'll give me a glimmer of hope that, maybe I will have a chance to fight the cancer, perhaps even beat it. Even if I didn't believe it I had to be strong for my wife and sons.

During this wait time the Sochi Olympics are taking place in Russia. I watched the Olympics as much as I could to keep myself occupied, to keep my thoughts from the upcoming oncologist visit and from the cancer growing inside me slowly killing me. I think that these will be the last Olympics I'll ever see. There were occasions I felt like I was floating in the air above the armchair looking down at myself.

I was scared, helpless. I was going to die. SOON. I would cry when alone. I would try to stay strong, positive. No one can understand the feelings, emotions, and fear your feeling. You close your eyes and the fear gets worse. You open your eyes and the fear becomes reality. There is no relief, no safe place to go to. The fight was becoming unbearable. I reached a point where I felt I couldn't do it anymore. Maybe I should accept faith and give up. It would be easier who could blame me. Fighting is hard but I had to at least try.

The day of the oncologist appointment arrives. Once again, I couldn't slow down time. I sat in the waiting room with Darlene unable to believe I would soon learn if I was going to live or die. That reality struck me harder than a brick in the face when my name was called. Yet again we're waiting in another room. This time it's small and confining and I feel suffocated.

My oncologist walks in with my file in her hands. In essence with my life in her hands. She reviews the medical report which signals my official death sentence. The February CT Scan confirms the colon cancer has spread to my liver and both lungs. Worse, the tumors have grown since my surgery almost two months prior. She said other things I didn't hear because I'd entered shutdown mode. My brain had automatically cut off all sound. My life was over. When I finally came back to reality, I asked the oncologist if I had inoperable liver cancer. She replied "yes". The one word at that precise moment in time I dreaded and despised the most. She continued to land the final blow. I have approximately six months of life remaining. Six months normally is not a long time but now that was all the time I had left to live. She advised that since the cancer was in my liver and both lungs, I may want to get my affairs in order. She informed me that I would begin "comfort chemo" in late February to help me deal with the pain and discomfort.

"Comfort Chemo!" What's comforting about injecting toxic poisons into your body when you've been told it won't keep you alive? It will only cause side effects that eventually ravage an already ravaged body. Was I wrong to feel this way? Who knows? I certainly didn't have the answer, not then, not now.

Darlene and I left the clinic deflated and filled with despair. I realized all hope was gone. All attempts at positivity were at an end. I was tired of deceiving myself and my family. The moment had come to accept my fate and make funeral arrangements. How would I tell my mother with failing health that she was going to lose another child? How could I tell my sons?

We break the news to our boys. Their response shocked and surprised me yet made me proud. They responded with the same message my wife had said on our way home from the clinic. "The fight begins now. You are not giving up. You have the three of us. We are in this together." These words stayed with me during the long months of struggling to battle an enemy intent on winning the war at any cost. I kept the truth from my mother as long as I could. When she found out she was stronger than I had given her credit for. My mother said "Bob my son we will fight this together. I will be there for you. Don't you give up."

I decided that very day not to give up. I had to show my wife and more importantly my sons that you never fold and give in no matter what life throws at you. They hadn't given up, neither could I. As long as there is a breath in your body you can fight. Darlene would often quote a line from my favorite movie Shawshank Redemption – "Get busy living or get busy dying". I was determined to get busy living, to be as normal as possible. I had to try to enjoy whatever time was left to me until that wasn't possible anymore.

Before beginning chemotherapy, my son Bobby told his mother about research he'd done on hash oil. How it claimed to cure cancer patients. I was doubtful about the purported results. Still, perhaps that was a ray of hope I needed. Hash oil wasn't recognized by the medical profession. If I disclosed the use of hash oil, there was a real possibility the oncologist would refuse to treat me. Therefore, I kept it a secret. For the next two years, Darlene and my sons extracted hash oil from weed. I'd take it three times a day during the entirety of my twenty-four chemotherapy treatments. By the time chemo was over I had consumed approximately sixty grams of hash oil. I would suggest if you contemplate using it for medical reasons do the research and make your own decision.

4
———

YOU WIN SOME, YOU LOSE SOME

M y first round of chemotherapy is scheduled for late February two months after my colon surgery. I have already started taking the hash oil which I hoped and prayed would help.

Before the chemo begins, I sit through a half-day session in the Chemo Unit to discuss what will happen during the treatments. They talk about the drugs I'll receive. They give us a kit to use at home composed of a HazMat suit and materials to use in case of a chemo spill. Family members would have to leave while you clean up. I take a cognitive test to affirm whether or not I have the mental capability to sign the approval form to receive chemo. As an aside, I must admit I cheated. When I was asked a question, the nurse gave me time to think about the answer while she went to the other patient to ask him a question. While she was doing this, I'd write the answer on my hand so I wouldn't forget. This was one test I had to pass.

They explain the process to follow if I have a chemo reaction while at home. A chemo bottle will be attached to me intravenously through a port which is inserted under the skin of my chest. For three more days at home after my chemo treatment at the hospital more toxic drugs are pumped into my body. When the three days have passed, I'll go to the public health nurse, who will be dressed in a protective HazMat suit to have the empty bottle removed from the port in my chest.

This session really set me back. I couldn't believe what lay ahead for me. The other man in attendance was visibly shocked as well. Just like me, he did not want to be there. The nurse asked if we had any questions. The man said, quite sorrowfully, that all he wanted was to go home. I never did find out if he survived.

The following week I walked into the Cancer Clinic for my first treatment. I was so stunned and in shock I wasn't able to speak. Darlene had to register for me. Previously, whenever I passed by the Cancer Clinic to visit family or friends in the hospital, I'd feel sorry for those who had to take that dreaded left turn into the Cancer Unit. I'd reflect on how lucky I was not to be going in there. Now, here I am taking that left turn. What happened? How did I arrive at this point? I still don't believe it. I just want to go home to my safe place. I knew I couldn't. My one and only chance to live was to stay and take these horrible drugs. I'm sure my wife experienced the same doubts and worries. But she never showed it.

The cancer clinic pharmacy won't mix your cocktail of drugs until you register at the desk. They will never pre-order them because of the cost of the drugs and the fear the patient won't show up. If this happened they would have to dispose of the bio-hazardous waste (Yes! Chemotherapy drugs are considered bio-hazardous waste).

I sat with Darlene waiting for my name to be called. Everyone in this room looks weak, but mostly sad. I wonder to myself how many of them will survive. What type of cancer do they have? Is this their first treatment? One lesson Darlene taught me was never compare yourself or whatever it is you are suffering from to another person. She would say every person, every illness is different. The will to fight, the will to survive, is different in every person. In my case I was dealing with cancer. I had to find that will to fight, that will to survive. You have to find your own inner strength. Just because someone lost their fight that doesn't mean you are going to lose yours.

Two hours later my specific combination of drugs are mixed, and I'm called into the treatment room. As I walk to my assigned chemo chair, I glance around. The room is filled to capacity with people of all ages and both sexes. Cancer spares no one. This is the one place I never thought I'd be. Cancer happens to others. Not to me. I start to pity myself. Sudden panic and fear engulfs me, overtakes me. I want to run out of this horrendous place. This can't be real. Will I be able to sit still long enough to undergo the procedure?

I recognize the woman sitting next to me as she's from my childhood neighborhood. She must see the fear on my face and tells me she had colon cancer and it had spread to her liver. She tells me this is her third treatment and talks about her cancer journey. Then she describes what I'm about to undergo. Her treatments have been slow because she's had bad reactions such as low blood count and infections. At that time, I didn't realize there could be such severe reactions. I guess you could say I was a rookie and wasn't prepared to hear what she told me. In retrospect it did help me prepare myself for the first round. The lady was going through a difficult time yet wanted to help me. I never forgot her kindness and always tried to help the "rookies" on their first day in the Chemo Unit.

She helps me understand things could go seriously bad with treatment and that I had to arrive with the right attitude. I had to prepare myself both mentally and physically to receive the dreadful yet life-saving drugs. I must accept that this unit is the best place for me, and I need to make it work.

My drugs arrived in a red box. It could just as easily be someone bringing your lunch, except the bearer is dressed in a HazMat suit for their own protection. The nurse, also wearing a HazMat suit signs for the box. She hooks the bag up to me the same way they hook you to an intravenous line. My blood pressure is extremely elevated, and the nurse reassures me that's normal for anyone undergoing their first injection.

I'm in distress. My heart is racing so fast I'm afraid I'll pass out. Yet the nurse doesn't appear concerned. I guess that this is routine for her. In a strange way, her calm demeanor and easy attitude settled me down. I'm unable to explain the despair that rushed over me the instant the nurse rolled the intravenous line clip and the drugs started to flow. I looked at Darlene. We both knew there was no turning back. Death or life starts right here and right now.

When chemo is finished I take home a portable bottle with additional chemo attached to my chest. I'm also prescribed steroids for the next three days which help control the nausea, vomiting and diarrhea. The steroids give you energy. Your heart races and you want to enjoy these three days of freedom. On the fourth day the sickness and exhaustion hits with full force. If only the steroids could be taken for the next eleven days before treatment time came around again. The doctors had told me I was going to die so why not let me take them for the duration between treatments. Now, I do understand why athletes take steroids to recover more quickly from an injury.

The steroids gave me energy. The hash oil helped with the nausea and sickness. The hash oil also helped me sleep and experts agree that sleep helps you heal. I'm not recommending hash oil as a treatment for cancer. I know it helped me, in that it eased nausea and sickness and allowed me the precious sleep I craved and needed.

My first treatment went well, no real problems to speak of. I received a combination of seven drugs. The take home chemo bottle was attached before I left. After the third day I went to the local Community Health Clinic to have it removed by a nurse dressed in a HazMat suit. These drugs are dangerous to a healthy person, and I wonder what they must be doing to my body. What a feeling of relief to be free from that bottle!

I have chemo treatments every two weeks for twenty-four weeks which amounted to twelve treatments. A port was inserted inside my upper right chest. This is an easier and better system to receive the chemo, as opposed to being hooked up to an intravenous line through a needle in my arm. I hated the idea of having a port and the night before the procedure I couldn't sleep. It scared me to have a foreign object inside my body. I tried to understand the fear I was feeling, and in thinking back I realized it was due to the fact everything I was going through was real and not a dream.

My second treatment went okay. Once the three days of taking steroids is over you begin to feel the power of the drugs: nausea, vomiting, exhaustion. Around the eleventh day the symptoms ease. Then, three days later you have the next treatment, and the process starts all over again.

Round four of my chemo brings a different result. I

begin to lose my taste. The food I once enjoyed now tastes like sulfur. No wonder the pounds fall off you as you don't want to eat. Not because you can't eat due to sickness, at least in my case, but because all food tastes like rotten eggs. Oddly, yet lucky for me I could taste Rice Crispy cereal along with A & W hamburgers. As well, I could taste and enjoy Mick and Sandy's beef soup that Sandy faithfully cooked for me and kept me well supplied. By day eleven my taste would return. Then day fourteen and another treatment bringing on nausea, vomiting, diarrhea, and exhaustion. The cycle repeats itself over and over. I hated this but what else could I do. I had to believe, to keep hoping the toxic drugs were helping. Even though the oncologist called it comfort chemo you must have hope. If you lose it there's nothing left to cling to. It's now April 2014. Nothing has changed. I have four months to live. The reality of that thought hits me hard!

I was going through chemo treatments and told I had little chance of survival. I began to wonder if the torment, the chemo, the constant sickness was worth it. Maybe it would be better to just lie down and give up. My wife and sons would not let that happen. My sister Linda would always say she had this feeling that everything would work out for me and that I would beat this dreaded disease. My wife, sons or my sister couldn't understood the emotions, the feelings, the fear I was going through. They weren't facing death in the face. I had four months to live. Fighting took away all the energy I had left in me. I wanted to fight but I also wanted to make the most of the months I had left to live. I had to at least give it a chance, if not for me at least for them.

It's April 8th, 2014 and I've lived to see another birthday. I would look at my family and cry when they were not there. I was devastated, in complete disbelief my life was about to end. The strain of what was happening to me caused my voice to fade. I had my family around me but I felt alone. Alone in the fact that I was dying. We are all going to die but when you are given just months to live the fear and emotions you feel are indescribable.

I've had four rounds of chemo and feel miserable. I continue to take the hash oil, and I'm convinced it's enabled me to sleep which in turn helps me maintain my energy. I try to stay positive and continue the fight if not for me but for my family. It's Sunday April 20th, 2014. Darlene and I decide to go for a drive to our cabin. My wife drives as she has been doing since my treatments. The drive to the cabin takes about one hour, half way there I have a sudden sharp pain in my right lower calf muscle. The road to the cabin is blocked with snow so we're forced to go by foot. I become stuck in a snowbank and can't move. Darlene is ahead of me and hears me calling to her. I laugh and say this is not the way I thought I would die.

My heart is racing as I'm trying with my wife's help to move forward, to get out of this predicament. The struggle is so severe I forget about the pain in my right leg. My heart is literally beating out of my chest. I manage to extricate myself. I realize the pain is gone. By now I'm exhausted, even though the cabin is a few yards away it takes me another five minutes to reach it.

Once inside I joke with my wife that we should make love as this may be our last chance. I'm not sure why I thought this. Maybe it's the hash oil talking. Darlene made the excuse it was too cold. (Was she thinking of me or her?) Oh well, I thought to myself at least I tried. We sat in the sun room, looking out at the pond and the surrounding hills. We leave the cabin a few hours later. The pain in my calf hadn't returned and I didn't give it any more consideration.

Three days later I had another CT scan to check if the cancer had spread. The oncologist routinely checked for one of two things: the cancer had gotten smaller and/or the cancer remained the same size. Darlene and I left the hospital, once again thinking about the wait for the results. The CT technician called our cell phone as we were pulling out of the hospital parking lot. My heart immediately beat out of my chest as panic set in. I believed this couldn't be good news thinking the treatment had failed and the cancer has spread like wildfire.

The technician said something has shown up in the scan and I'm to go to the ER immediately. I pressed for more information, but the technician repeated to get back to the hospital. Darlene parked the car and we rushed to the ER. She explained to the triage nurse we had received a call from the CT technician telling us to get to the ER as soon as possible. The triage nurse calmly told us to take a seat in the waiting room. I paced for forty-five minutes in a state of constant panic. It's a miracle I didn't have a heart attack.

My wife, a usually laid back, respectful person felt we had waited long enough and spoke once more to the nurse. This time in a rather forceful tone of voice and in no uncertain terms she told the nurse that I had been ordered to the ER immediately, and not to waste time. Why have we been forced to wait for almost an hour to find out why?

This time the nurse appeared to grasp the seriousness of my situation and immediately brought us inside. The doctor came in looking utterly taken aback which quite frankly surprised me. He inquired if I knew the reason I'd been told to report to the ER. At first, I was amused by the question and responded. Sure, I have cancer and just had a CT scan.

They called and ordered me here. I thought, haven't you read the triage nurse's report. The doctor's next words floored me. "We can't believe you walked in here. You should be dead." Darlene and I stared at each other. Did we really hear that! Darlene fell back in her chair, speechless.

I finally found my voice and said, "I'm not feeling great, but not any worse than the last four months."

The doctor quickly clarified the situation. "The CT scan shows you have two blood clots. One passed through your heart from your lungs and the other one is currently wrapped around your liver." He went on to say that blood clots kills seventy-five percent of people on the spot. Of the twenty-five percent who survive the initial onset of one blood clot, half of those die in the ambulance on the way to the hospital. I had two! Yet again I'm not sure why I survived. The doctors immediately put me on blood thinners.

A short while later a female doctor arrives and she asks me. If I go into "distress (vital signs aren't detectable) do I want to be resuscitated?" She sounded mechanical. My wife and I are shocked and rather disgusted by the question. Darlene delivers the answer to her in no uncertain terms. "You better believe he does."

I expressed to the doctor that I was not impressed with her question, particularly at this period in my life. I explained to her I had four months left to live. Every second, every minute, every hour is important to me. I wouldn't be here if I wasn't fighting to live. She replied that she was only doing her job. When she left, an ER nurse who'd overheard the exchange came in and thanked us for standing up to this doctor who had asked that question many times before at the most vulnerable and frightening times of a patient's life and had never been challenged.

Later that evening at 9:00 P.M. something miraculous happened. The ER doctor comes into my room and discusses with myself and Darlene my cancer diagnosis, the CT scan, and the earlier call to come back to the hospital. Most of all he was interested in talking about the blood clots as he was flabbergasted I'd survived without any obvious adverse side effects. He wanted to know what I had done over the past few days. I told him about the trip to the cabin, the pain in my calf and being stuck in the snowbank. He wasn't positive but felt getting stuck in the snow may have saved my life. My heart beating so rapidly may have forced the clot through my lungs and heart. He was still awed that I was alive and even more miraculously sitting up and talking.

Unexpectedly he asked if I had the results of the CT scan. I said no that I had an appointment scheduled for next week with the oncologist. He had the results and said that he was surprised and unable to explain what has happened. If only I could control my morbid thoughts and keep my heart from racing. Of course, I'm expecting to hear the worst possible news.

The doctor opens the report and reads that all five spots on the right side of my liver measuring five centimeters each have shrunk to five millimeters each. He was confounded as I'd only had four chemo treatments to date. Darlene and I cried. For the first time we believed I had a real chance to beat this horrible disease. The doctor however added that there weren't any changes in my lung tumors which I took as good news. They hadn't grown! I wondered to myself if the hash oil had played a part in the miraculous shrinkage. What a day! I survived life-threatening blood clots and now I found hope, real hope that I'd been searching for, praying for. I had a real chance at life. It's amazing how quick you can go from death to life. Once again my dreams and plans returned. But as they did I thought could this news be a mistake? This has happened to me before. I asked the doctor to recheck the report and make sure what he was telling us was indeed the correct assessment. I take nothing for granted anymore. He reassures my wife and I that the tumors have indeed shrunk.

I spent overnight in the ER. The next day my oncologist visited me and immediately prescribed a stronger blood thinner called Lovonox. She released me from the hospital much later in the day with enough Lovonox for a few weeks. Before I leave another group of doctors speak to me with the news that the blood clots have damaged the right side of my heart. Like I said before. You win some. You lose some. They assure me the damage will heal over time. Another shock thrown my way and I think let's put that issue aside as I have more pressing things to worry about. Besides, mentally I couldn't carry another burden.

The day of the appointment with my oncologist arrives. As I walk down the stairs to the clinic, I recall all that's happened to me during the week. The blood clots, heart damage, the liver tumors shrinking, the spots on my lungs remaining the same. I try to remain positive but the negative thoughts creep in like intruders breaking into your home at night. The clinic is full of patients of all ages, gender, and ethnicity. Cancer doesn't discriminate. It occurs to me I'm no different than anyone else. They must feel as I do, in disbelief they're fighting the battle for their very lives. Suddenly, I no longer pity myself. I used to think "why me?" Now I think "why not me?"

From the waiting area you're escorted into a smaller inner waiting room where the walls are lined with images of different types of cancer, not something you really want to see at that point. There's a slight tap on the door and the oncologist walks in. She explains the results of my CT scan adding that she's blown away by my incredible shrinking tumors. She hadn't expected this outcome and now will change her approach to my treatment by getting more aggressive, no more "comfort chemo." However she never addressed her initial assessment that my life was approaching the end and I never asked in fear of the answer. I was disappointed. I had thought if the tumors had shrunk doesn't that give me a chance to beat this cancer.

Of course, she asks if I'm taking any other source of treatment that she's not aware of. I keep the hash oil to myself for fear she may refuse further treatment. We then discuss the blood clots. She's amazed I survived and tells me a person with cancer undergoing chemo therapy is susceptible to blood clots. As she is talking, I'm wondering why I wasn't automatically prescribed a blood thinner as a precaution. Perhaps there's a medical reason which she doesn't explain. Then again I didn't ask.

She decides to keep me on the Lovonox for the time being and gives me a prescription which costs approximately $1,200 a month. Thankfully my insurance covered the cost of the drug. I enquired about those who didn't have insurance, what did they do? I was surprised and happy to hear the clinic has the means to pay for those who can't afford to pay themselves.

I left the oncologist office disappointed that I hadn't received the news I had expected. That now I had a chance to live. My wife as usual had a different view of our meeting with the doctor. She commented to me that she wouldn't be changing my course of treatment if she didn't believe I had a chance. I listened to my wife, what she said made sense. I took her view of the meeting. My wife looks at the positive and always looks for the good news. We should all have her sense of optimism. What a better world this would be if we looked at life like my wife does.

Lovonox turns out to be a liquid drug which has to be injected into my torso twice a day. It was difficult at first, but I soon got the hang of it. There were days I forgot to inject myself. Darlene would remind me by coming to the living room smiling as she waved the needle in front of me. We laughed each time this happened. There were times when I purposely "forgot" to inject myself just so we could have a good laugh. Yep, even suffering with cancer you can still find joy in the small things.

Since my tumors had shrunk, the word "comfort" was dropped from the name of the treatments. The biweekly chemo treatment continued along with blood tests and monthly CT scans. I'd see the oncologist before each treatment and a week following a CT scan. June 2014 came, five months since I was told I had six months to live. I wasn't feeling great but at least I was still alive. I now had hope; I now believed that just maybe I could beat this horrible disease. I decided to focus on life not on death.

My wife accompanied me on each and every test and appointment, she never missed one. Months went by and my wife and I and my sons continued the fight. She always sensed when I was feeling down, depressed, or the numerous occasions I wanted to give up. There were many times when the nausea, diarrhea, anger, frustration, and chemo brain confusion, eroded my will to fight. Darlene, a five-foot two woman was and still is my rock, the support that she gave me, a six-foot two man; she gave me the desire to keep going. She was my strength, she kept me alive. When at my lowest she'd order me into our car and take me for a drive or we'd go to a movie. She'd always think of an activity to keep me busy in order to keep my mind off my condition.

When I began taking the hash oil, my son Bobby was the one who prepared it until he trained his mother in the process. One ounce of weed produces a batch of oil which lasts for two weeks. The weed has to be cooked on the stove top to bring out the oil. On one particular day Darlene and Bobby had left the kitchen for a moment while the hash cooked. I'll blame what I did next on my "chemo brain." I turned up the heat on the burner, and within seconds the oil caught on fire with smoke billowing from the frying pan. I tried to douse it with a towel with no luck, spreading the flame to the floor. Oh no, I thought, the house was going to burn down. I yelled at Darlene to get out, to save herself and call the fire department. Bobby grabbed a fire extinguisher and had the fire out in seconds. In a flash, $300 of weed had truly gone up in smoke. I didn't even get to inhale the smoke and take a trip.

Due to my stupidity the kitchen flooring had to be replaced and the walls and ceiling repainted. There was no way we would call the insurance and tell them I started the fire cooking hash oil. Even going through chemo and with the help of my boys we completed the renovations on our own. This difficult work exhausted me. I'd become frustrated not being able to work as efficiently as I used to and would sit on the floor with my head in my hands. Tigi, our Pitbull would join me. Her very presence was calming. I tried to be as normal as possible, it was hard but you have to try.

Josh still lived at home with us, and he'd been assigned the job of keeping me physically active. He walked Tigi every day and insisted I come along. Dad, he'd say. If you're not up to walking stay in the truck and wait for us.

My son knows his father well. His strategy worked. I always forced myself to walk with him and Tigi. We'd drive to the dirt road that leads to the hill where there's a water tower at the top surrounded by a fence with a gate at its centre. My goal was to reach that gate. Josh would park at the bottom of the hill. Each day I made it a little further. I'd never look at the gate as I walked because it would discourage me to see the distance left to travel. Even though the distance wasn't that far, it was a daunting task. I'd have difficulty breathing and forced to stop after a few hundred feet.

This continued for months as I was making it a little further each day. Three months into this I decided I was going to make it to the dam gate. The many days and weeks of pacing myself paid off. I made it to the gate along with Josh and Tigi. I was so proud to achieve the goal I'd set for myself, I did the "Rocky" dance. By setting small goals and sticking to them I touched the gate. I saw the pride in my son's eyes and knew in that moment he'd also won a victory.

What a sense of accomplishment filled me! Even Tigi sensed it for she jumped around even more excited than Josh and me. I connected with Josh in a special way that day. He fought the actual uphill battle with me intent on never giving up. This day is a win for me in more than one way. Hopefully there would be many more to come.

Darlene and I continue the daily drives and movie day. We even went on short walks. During one of these walks in the park I slipped and fell down. I tried to get to my feet but couldn't. I looked up at Darlene with tears in my eyes and said, "Honey, I can't get up. I don't have the strength." People passed by as if we didn't exist which was unusual. Perhaps they thought I was intoxicated. Thinking about that incident I can see their point of view. I'm haggard looking, feeble, and attempting to stand up. Haven't we all seen a drunken person in that state?

My short petite wife gathers up all her strength and finally manages to help me up. It amazes me how she managed it. Before cancer, at six feet two I weighed 235 pounds. I now weigh 190. My wife held on to me as I stumbled back to the car. It was one of the most humbling and degrading days of my cancer journey. I had always been physically strong and able to care for myself. Yet here I was lying on the ground unable to gather enough strength to pick myself up. Once home I sat in the armchair and cried. I felt useless, hurt at what I'd become. It was the lowest point in my struggle.

The last few treatments had worn me down physically and mentally, my will to fight was fading and then the fall in the park. That was the straw, as they say that broke me. I had enough. No one could blame me for giving up. I'd tried and tried and tried and was just too tired to go on. Mentally I was overburdened. I wanted this to be over. I was ready to die, to be at peace, to have all the worry gone, over. No more chemotherapy. No more CT scans. No more meeting with the oncologist. I was ready to give up. I had enough. I wanted this to be over. I wanted more than anything for my wife and boys to understand. I had fought the good fight, but the time had come to accept my fate and allow death to happen.

As the tears fell and these thoughts consumed me Josh walked into the room. I don't want him to see me like this and quickly brush away the tears. One glance at my face he knew all the emotions ripping away inside me. "Dad," he said. "I believe you need a hug." When he put his arms around me all the sorrow and morbid thoughts evaporated. He gave me the courage to fight on. Once again Josh saved my life. You win some. You lose some. I considered my fall a loss. Josh turned it into a win.

I look at my boys and try to imagine what they must think and feel watching their father die, watching their father waste away, watching their father fight, yet appear to be losing the battle. What fears are now ingrained in their minds about their future health? Dad had prostate and bowel cancer. Now he has liver and lung cancer. Will we end up with these cancers? Has our chances for this increased? I do my best to turn their fears into a positive by explaining they'll have to be tested sooner than normal. If there's an issue it will be dealt with, for early detection is the key to success, the key to survival. The cancer won't have spread like mine had.

I hasten to add they won't necessarily be diagnosed with cancer because I was. Worried for my sons I spoke to the oncologist about their risk for prostate cancer. She explains that all men have a ten percent chance of getting prostate cancer. My sons' chances rise fifty percent of the ten percent which means their chance of prostate cancer rises to fifteen percent. The same percentage applies to colon cancer. Bobby and Josh were relieved to hear this. The odds are slightly increased, thus the requirement for early testing. They promised me they'd get tested early.

I was nearing the last of my twelve chemo treatments. With each treatment I grew more fatigued and took longer to recover. My energy level and strength were draining away. Dressing in the morning had become a major challenge. My will to fight was waning and I preferred to stay home. Darlene and the boys would not allow that. They did everything in their power to lift my spirits. I continued to take the hash oil and go on the walks with Josh and Tigi. All I wanted to do was to lie down and to be left alone. My taste was gone and didn't return on day eleven as before. The CT scans continued and the tumors on my liver remained at five millimeters which I took as good news. Further shrinkage was preferred, yet not growing either was considered a win.

It's July 2014 and I've completed my last round of chemo. I meet with my oncologist and she explains she is going on maternity leave and would be forwarding my file onto another oncologist. Since chemo treatments had concluded, I asked what are the next steps in my course of treatment. She said I'll be watched to see if the tumors had changed, as chemotherapy remains in your system for a while and continues to destroy cancer cells. She talked about a committee of surgeons who review files sent to them by oncologists to determine if surgery is viable or to offer other treatment options. However, she felt in my case, my cancer was too far advanced. She said there's nothing they could do for me. I thought, why did she bring up this committee if I had no chance of survival? Despite the oncologist's dire statement, I decided then and there not to give up. Another CT scan was scheduled as well as an appointment to meet the new oncologist in late July.

5

AN UNEXPECTED TURN OF EVENTS!

During chemotherapy I made many friends in the unit. You sit next to them for hours at a time while you're being pumped full of toxic drugs. How can you not get close to people going through an emotional and physical upheaval? Each person had an impact on me which still lingers to this day. My heart went out to each and every person.

The nurses, who work there are the best of their profession. They were caring and understood our needs and most of all our fears and treated us with the utmost dignity and respect. They get to know you and your family. Their patients are fighting this dreadful disease and they know some will lose their battle. They have to remain unattached. But let's be real, they're only human. Working in this environment with patients they have gotten close to dying, has to affect them.

Some people tolerate chemotherapy, others have reactions such as low white blood cell levels or infections which can result in delayed treatment or even discontinuation of treatment indefinitely. The lady from my childhood neighborhood, who I sat next to for my first treatment didn't make it. I'd finished round twelve and she hadn't made it to round five before she died. She was in her early fifties. I felt so sad for her husband and family. Learning of her passing really set me back, but I knew I couldn't let it get me down. I had to keep going.

A gentleman I'd worked with came into the clinic for his first treatment while I was receiving my last. He sat in his chemo chair waiting for his treatment to begin. I saw in his eyes that he was sad, lost, completely bewildered. When I approached him, he could barely speak. It seems we all have the same reaction when first faced with cancer and the thought of chemotherapy. His wife told me he had bowel cancer which had spread. The same cancer as I had. I tried offering him advice on what to expect. I tried to give him hope, something to cling to. It was obvious to me he wasn't in the frame of mind to hear anything I or anyone else had to say.

I understood what he was going through even though it's hard I firmly believe that's the time you need to listen to the stories of hope, stories of survival, and to drown out the stories of death, drown out the negative people and surround yourself with those who really care. I left that last chemo treatment thinking about my ex-coworker and praying that he'd pull through.

Less than two months later, Darlene and I were having lunch in a restaurant when the wife of my ex-coworker stopped by our table to say hello. I asked how her husband was doing and she answered by saying, "You haven't heard?" From her response I knew what she would say next. She told me he had died a few weeks earlier. She told us he became tired. He was in so much pain. He had tried to fight but it became too much for him. I didn't know what to say. How do you console someone who's lost their life partner to a devastating, unrelenting disease? I felt guilty because I was still alive. I couldn't look at her as she sat at the table across from us.

There are many more such stories I could tell. I realize how hard cancer patients fight to live and how difficult it is for family members to watch that struggle. I decide that day in the restaurant that if I focus on death, I'll lose my sense of life and the will to fight for it. Therefore, I have to move past the sadness and despair I'm feeling. I try to park these stories as they will certainly bring me to a place I can't go to at this time in my journey. You must stay positive. Every person's story is different. Every cancer is different. This is the message Darlene constantly reinforced when I heard about people dying from cancer. From that day at the restaurant whenever she heard of another cancer death, she kept it from me.

The time to learn the results of my July 2014 CT scan had arrived. I'd finished all twelve treatments and would learn if the tumors had shrunk any further. As usual, anxiety, fear and panic come with it. My thoughts run wild yet again. If nothing's changed or worse then what? Is that the end for me? Do I now have to start planning for my death? Nothing that's said can push those thoughts away. All that's left for me is to hope for the best outcome. This scared me. If only I could slow down time. Unfortunately, these are the occasions where time speeds up.

Darlene and I are outside the Oncologist's office, in a room filled with patients. Little did I know I was her last appointment of the day. Finally, I'm called in only to be seated in that ten-by-ten windowless room where those cancer pictures line the walls. We wait for what seems like hours to me but is actually a few minutes. My heart rate and thoughts are in overdrive. I'm shaking all over. Panic has me in a strangle hold. I see the shadows of people walking by the office through the bottom of the door. Every sound from outside induces more anxiety in me. Has the cancer grown? My chemo was over, if nothing changed on the CT scan then what? I thought if the scan shows no improvement then I guess that's it I'm done. I had nothing left to grab on to, I was petrified. All these thoughts and feelings accost you while sitting in this small room, waiting for a sentence of either death or life.

There's a light tap on the door and in walks the replacement Oncologist. She introduces herself. Her attitude is friendly and upbeat. Is this a sign of good news? She explains my tumors haven't changed since the previous scan. Then she drops a bombshell. My original oncologist had sent my file to the surgical review committee before leaving for maternity leave. I wasn't sure I'd heard correctly and interrupted the oncologist to ask her to repeat what she'd said. She confirms that my file had been sent to the review committee. This was a complete and total shock and I asked how this happened. She explained that my Oncologist had decided to send the file just to give me a chance, even though she wasn't entirely confident of it making a difference. She felt that with more eyes reviewing my case they may have a different opinion. Thank God she sent my file. Thank God she gave me this opportunity. For that I will always be grateful to her.

The oncologist went on to say the majority of the committee agreed there was nothing they could do for me. However, two young surgeons were more optimistic in the possibility that they could do something. They wanted to meet with me to discuss surgery and to give their opinion concerning my chances of survival and my willingness to proceed. They would then review my case in more detail. If one of them decided against surgery the other would as well. It was an all or nothing scenario. They reasoned if the liver was inoperable there was no sense operating on the lungs since the liver cancer would kill me. Both surgeons had to agree to proceed with surgery.

The Oncologist gave me the names of the two surgeons and said it was my responsibility to contact them and arrange appointments. The one thing I would recommend to all the doctors out there would be to never dash a patient's hope. Leave them with at least a glimmer of optimism, a glimmer of hope. Sometimes that's all that is needed. The rest is up to the patient. I'd been granted another win even though it could just as easily become a loss. I had that ray of hope I was looking for. Once again, I had a chance to get my life back, to get my dreams back. I was overwhelmed with joy but cautious not to get too optimistic. I had to stay calm. Another let down could destroy my will to fight and take away whatever hope I had left.

As it was late in the day Darlene called both surgeons the next morning. She first spoke to the doctor who would perform the liver surgery. I received an appointment to see him for mid-September 2014 which was in six weeks' time. Surgery couldn't even be considered until six weeks following my last chemo treatment. The appointment for the lung surgeon was scheduled for a week after I'd seen the liver surgeon.

Those six weeks were tough to endure. Once I wanted time to slow down now I wished it would speed up. I was confused and scared because my life hung in the air. Religion wasn't an important aspect in my life in terms of going to church and all that it entails. When you're facing what was in store for me you search for a higher power. I'd ask

God to protect my family and bring me good health. My once a month visit to the local church continued and I would pray for my family and ask for help to get through what was to come my way.

I tried to carry on a normal life during those six weeks. Walks and movie nights with my wife. Walks with Josh and Tigi. I continued taking the hash oil. My taste returned and it was fantastic to enjoy my favorite foods such as turkey dinner, fish and chips and toast in the morning. No more Rice Crispy cereal. I even gained a little weight.

Six weeks later Darlene and I wait to meet the liver surgeon in a small windowless room with those same cancer pictures all around us. Darlene quietly tells me not to talk about what he might or might not say. Don't dwell on the worst case scenarios so we can prepare ourselves for bad news. As she is saying this a young surgeon comes in with my file. He has an air of confidence which I find reassuring. He introduces himself and comes straight to the point. He has reviewed my case and believes he can operate. The tumors are situated on the right side of my liver. Apparently the possibility of surgery is greatly improved when the cancer is on the right side.

However there's one unexpected problem. The left side of my liver is smaller than the right with the right being seventy percent of the total. The left side has to be fifty percent before he can operate. He explained that years ago this would have totally eliminated surgery. Today there is a procedure which fools the left side of the liver into believing the right side has died. The left will grow to compensate for the loss. He added there's no guarantee the procedure will work for me but there has been a high rate of success. I eagerly replied, "Let's do this."

He then asked if I had scheduled a meeting with the

lung surgeon. If lung surgery wasn't possible, he wouldn't perform his surgery, thus the scheduling of the procedure to enlarge my liver was dependent upon the lung surgeon's decision to operate or not. I promised to get back to him as soon as I had the second surgeon's opinion.

The doctor acknowledged that he was well acquainted with the lung surgeon and had discussed my file during the surgical review committee meeting. He asked for permission to speak with the lung surgeon about our meeting. Both doctors were good friends and often went to lunch together. Of course, I said no problem. The meeting concluded and the doctor said "I am ready to do my job, now tell the lung surgeon it's time for him to do his." This comment made me confident that I was in good hands.

The next week it's time to meet the lung surgeon. Once again, I suffer the anxiety, the shaking, and the dreaded small, enclosed waiting room. He sees the anxiety, the fear and anticipation on my face and without hesitation gives me his news. "I heard from the liver surgeon. He's a go and so am I." Darlene looks at me. There's a real chance I may beat this damm cancer. There were no real assurances. Are there any truly real assurances in life? These two doctors had given me a lifeline, something to hang on to. I can't say it enough. Hope is vital when fighting for your life. No matter how dire the news search for even the slightest glimmer of hope and hold it close to your heart. Remember to gather those who you love and give you strength around you and walk away from those who bring you down.

I'd been told ten months earlier I would be dead in six months. I'd already beaten the odds and now was given another chance to beat the odds. Darlene and I have gone through a lifetime of hardship and worry. In the beginning you never know what you're capable of, but you know you have to fight. Giving up or giving in isn't a viable option. We have new obstacles to overcome. This time, however, we have the experience and the will to continue the fight. We have real hope. We have a real chance. I could feel life coming back inside me. The strain went out of my voice for the first time in almost a year. I began to once again have dreams about life and the things I thought I was going to miss.

A week later Darlene and I are in with the liver surgeon once again. He's spoken with the lung surgeon and he is now ready to do the first part of my liver surgery. He explains the procedure for enlarging my liver. A needle will be inserted into the right side of my upper torso to pinch off the main artery passing through the right side of the liver. The left side would believe the right side had died and would then grow to compensate for the loss. The success rate for this procedure was high and it would take eight weeks for the left side of the liver to grow. I saw this medical procedure as a true miracle of medicine. This procedure would give me a chance at life. Imagine if it didn't exist. Another lucky break, I wondered how many more would come my way.

I discovered on the day of the procedure that another doctor, with more expertise in this particular process, would perform the surgery. As I waited outside the operating room with Darlene a nurse came in to shave below the waist in preparation. I was confused as the needle would be inserted in the torso area. I told the nurse I'd prefer to shave myself and she handed over the razor. When she left, I passed it to Darlene. We both laughed as she handed it back to me. I'd just begun to shave when the doctor stepped in. He laughed and asked what I was doing. I explained and he laughed again saying, "The needle is going into your torso, not down there." The nurse apologized for the misunderstanding and we all laughed as she rolled me into the operating room. Humour really cuts through the anxiety.

The doctor told me he hoped to reach the artery on the first try but he said sometimes it can take several attempts. He said not to worry as he had done this many times before with success. I watched on the monitor as he inserted the needle, glad I was hooked up to pain medication. As the doctor pushed in the needle, I felt a severe pain in my right shoulder. Before the procedure I was instructed not to move but the pain was so intense.

My shoulder hurt because the artery in the liver is attached to the artery running through the shoulder to the neck. As he continued to push the needle in the pain intensified. I advised the doctor and he increased the pain medication, which didn't help. The pain intensified but I decided to tolerate it and not tell the doctor for fear he might stop the procedure. I got lucky as the doctor found the artery on the first try. I could see the doctor tie off the artery on the monitor. When he finished he told me all went well and he was optimistic that the left side of my liver would grow. He gave me the hope I was looking for. This procedure was the second most excruciatingly painful experience of my life, the first being that day in December when my family rushed me to the Emergency Room.

During the following eight weeks, I prayed and asked everyone I know to pray my liver would grow. The wait was difficult but by now I'm an old hand at waiting. This was one occasion I didn't want time to slow down. At the end of the eight weeks a CT scan is done. It's now December 2014 and the appointment with the liver surgeon has arrived. It's been a year since that fateful day I assumed I suffered from appendicitis. It's been ten months since I was given six months to live. The physical pain is difficult to take but the psychological pain is just as bad or maybe even worse.

Darlene and I were at the liver surgeon's office once again consumed with fear but this time I had a sense of optimism, maybe I had a real chance of survival. The surgeon walked in and wasted no time in conveying good news. The left side of my liver had grown to approximately fifty percent which in turn made surgery possible. He discussed the risks associated with such a surgery. I politely intervened to ask, "If I don't have the surgery what will happen?" He replied. "You will most likely die." I responded, "Then I don't need to hear the risks of surgery. Let's schedule it."

He explained he would have to remove my gall bladder in order to reach the liver. Once the right side was removed and the operation successful, the left side would continue to grow bringing my liver to a normal size. He scheduled the surgery for early March 2015 as he wanted to give my body time to regain strength from everything I'd been through for the past year. My chemo treatments were finished and I was terrified the liver and lung cancer would spread during the interim. I voiced my concern. The doctor insisted on the quoted waiting time. I understood he was the doctor and knew best.

Three surgeries lay ahead of me. One for the liver and one for each lung. I was scared however I viewed it as great news. This was a win and a renewed lease on life. We left the surgeons office feeling we had been given a chance to get our lives back. We decided to take the time before the surgery to just enjoy each other's company like we had done in the past. We would forget cancer and the surgeries ahead of me. We would spend time with our sons, make new memories. Everyone needed a break from cancer and the fight we had ahead of us.

My wife had been by my side since the first day of this journey. She never once let me see her sorrow. She never lost faith. She never got angry when I wanted to give up. She never complained. She never spoke about her own feelings of fear and despair. At times, I'd ask how she was holding up and always received the same answer that she was fine. Looking back I should have tried harder to understand what she was going through. I'm sure she cried when she was alone.

Darlene was strong, supportive, caring, and understanding. She made sure all my appointments were arranged and that I showed up on time. If I'd been on my own, I don't believe I would've had the strength to fight when all I wanted was to give up. I honestly believe her sheer force of will kept me alive during the bewildering cancer journey and she is the reason I'm alive today.

6

LIVER SURGERY

December 2014 to March 2015 I lived as normal a life as possible. Darlene and I briefly talked about a vacation but quickly put the idea aside so as not to jinx the upcoming surgery. Even though the future looked brighter fear managed to creep in. I'm lucky the three surgeries are a go, and as before the waiting game begins. After the liver and lung surgeries, it will take time for the tissue samples to be tested. Will all the cancer have been removed? If I dwell on the totality of all this, I'll panic. So, I make the choice to only think about the liver surgery for now. What benefit will it be to skip ahead?

My brother, Wayne visited while I contemplated all that lay ahead of me. He was a six-foot three fire fighter. Two years my senior. Shortly before my diagnosis in December 2013 we'd begun to reconnect as brothers and were on the way to becoming true friends. We had started dropping into each other's houses every now and again and we would talk about sports, politics, our lives, and our children. Then I got sick.

My sickness drew us closer. He seemed to show up when I needed him the most. When my liver operation was approaching, I was anxious, nervous. Sure enough, I'd see him coming through the front door. I confided all my fears about the surgery to him and how scared I was. He in turn related several of his many experiences as a firefighter which had brought on episodes of anxiety and depression. None of our siblings had any idea the tragedies he had witnessed and their lasting effects. He gave me a piece of advice, I remember and still use to this day. When you're overwhelmed, when panic sets in, when anxiety takes hold, close your eyes and in your mind go to a place where you feel the most relaxed and at peace. I take his advice and suddenly I'm sitting in my cabin's sunroom watching the sun set as it spreads its rays across the pond. I would take this imaginary journey often over the next three years.

It's early March 2015 and I'm at the hospital preparing for my liver surgery. My wife and sons are at my side. My mother and siblings are in the waiting room. God bless them. I love them now more than I ever did. They were there for me through those difficult frightening years and to this day I appreciate that.

The surgeon enters and begins to reiterate the pros and cons of the surgery. I interrupt saying, politely in a nervous voice, I understand the risk but I want to get on with surgery. He leaves saying "I'll see you in a few minutes."

I said good-bye to Darlene with the real possibility I might never see her again. Later I'm on the operating table with the doctor looking down at me. I'm hooked up to several machines and told to count backwards from ten. I believe I made it to seven. Six hours later I wake up in the Special Care Unit.

The nurse sees I'm awake and immediately informs the doctor. He tells me the surgery went well and the left side of my liver looked healthy. He tells me my gallbladder had a stone in it as big as the gallbladder itself. He'd never seen that before. It'll take about six to eight weeks for the liver to grow to full size. The right side of the liver and the gall bladder would be sent to the pathology laboratory for analysis. If the outside margins are free of cancer this will indicate the cancer hadn't spread to the left side of the liver or to other organs. I was so happy to wake up, I was still alive. Now to hear this great news. I was still worried about the tissue sample results but relieved I had one surgery over with and hopefully two more left.

Darlene and my boys were the only family permitted to visit me in the Special Care Unit. The doctor had already spoken to them about the surgery. A short while later when I was moved to a private room nausea kicked in. I felt so sick I was scared something was wrong and I was going to die. Two nurses sat by my side the whole night. I constantly vomited. They held tight to me to prevent my stiches from ripping open. The incision ran from the top of my chest in a semi-circle direction to my right hip. Pain doubled with each vomiting session. I was so weak I could hardly sit up in bed. I wouldn't have made it through the night without the help of those two wonderful caring nurses. By six a.m. I settled down and I fell asleep for a few hours.

It's a miracle my stiches didn't burst, or I hadn't damaged my liver that night. Before my surgery, I promised my wife I would get out of bed and walk the first morning after my surgery. That first morning I did indeed get up and started walking to the chair in the corner of the room. The nurse saw me and came running into my room and helped me get to the chair. I felt good about keeping my promise. The next night I couldn't sleep due to the constant noise of nurses walking by and patients crying out in pain. A man in another room constantly yelled and cursed the nurses. I was tempted to go to his room and have a strong word with him. I later learned he had several serious issues, and the nurses weren't upset with him, they understood. This incident taught me every person and every situation is different and you should never leap to a conclusion without all the facts. A philosophy I had normally followed in my life. I was tired and weak but still no reason to react like I did.

That same night I walked to the lobby at the far end of my floor and closed the door, thankful that I could drown out the sounds of sickness. My nurse was aware of where I had gone. For the next four nights I would sit in that lobby and take the imaginary journey to my cabin's sunroom, as my brother Wayne had advised.

On day five the surgeon visits pleased with my progress and that I've recovered faster than expected. He will be releasing me from hospital. He says I still have to wait for the report on my tissue samples. If the news isn't good there's nothing else that can be done for me. However, he is hopeful the biopsy results will be fine. The doctor schedules a follow-up appointment for early April as he should have the tissue results by then. I thanked him for his kindness and expertise. I had heard he was one of the top surgeons in the country and patients world-wide would request his services and expertise. Now I see why.

The thirty minutes I waited for Darlene to pick me up seemed like hours. While waiting, I try to remain positive, thinking everything will work in my favour, I've come too far now to hear bad news!

Driving home I confess that I'm worried about the lab results and moan, "When will we ever be free of this torment, of this constant worry?" For the first time since this journey began, Darlene replies sternly, "Bob, let's not go there. Look at how far you have come over the past months. Everything is going your way." She goes on to say, "we've overcome one hurdle, let's celebrate that victory, let's be happy for now."

I saw the happiness on her face and decided she was right. It was time I lifted her spirits. The past fifteen months had all been about me. She'd been through a hard time as well with no thought to herself. It was time to change that. I know how I felt physically and emotionally. What about her? I decided then and there to finally put Darlene's feelings ahead of mine for the first time. I promised not to complain. Not to voice my doubts. She deserved a break from having to constantly bear my burden as well as her own.

I managed this new resolve for about a week then the self-pity and self-worry took control once again. Nights were extremely taxing as the fears and concerns you keep at bay during the day hounded the dark hours. More terrifying were the weird dreams I experienced. I actually began to think I was going insane. The months of stress and worry had caught up with me. Sent me over the edge. I didn't know how to cope or who to turn to for help. I kept this from my wife and sons. I had to consider their feelings.

My brother, Wayne, visits and I tell him about the nightmares, about my fears and about how I'm feeling. He smiles and says, "Bob, you're having a reaction to the anesthetic they gave you during surgery." He understood about these things as having once been a paramedic in the fire department. He assured me these feelings would pass in a few days. I was so relieved I hugged him. The weird dreams and feelings ended as he predicted. He had an uncanny way of showing up at the precise moment I needed him the most.

During this period there weren't any side effects from the surgery. I was pain free and felt healthy. Even though I worried about my tissue results I remained hopeful. I'll repeat once again that one glimmer of hope is enough to keep you fighting. My mother lived in my basement apartment and dropped up often to see me. We'd talk about my childhood and the vacations she shared with my family. She had a look of sadness yet never spoke about the possibility of my death. In truth, she refused to accept such an eventuality.

Wayne, dropped by again to see me this time with tears in his eyes and he said to me, "I don't know how you do it, Bob, you were told you had six months to live. You were told you were going to die. Yet you fight on." He said he knew he wouldn't be able to handle news like that. I answered, no one knows how strong they are until they're faced with such news. Hopefully, you will never have to face that situation. If you do, I'm sure you will have the strength to face it. What choice do you have! When he left that day Darlene commented he didn't look well. He looked tired, like he had something on his mind. I should have sensed that something was off and asked how he was feeling. I never did and for that I am truly sorry.

My brothers and sisters often visited to inquire how I was feeling or if there was anything they could do for me. The conversations centered around the weather, sports, and their daily lives. They never asked how my wife was feeling or was there anything they could do for her. Most people focus on the person with the illness. It's important to never forget the partner and their suffering, their anguish. Inquire how they're doing, how are they coping. Darlene and I were left with all this anxiety and worry. I wished that for at least one day we could live with not a care in the world. That we could plan and talk about a vacation as my siblings did. Instead, we might never go on another trip. Never experience the joy of life again.

My siblings never truly understood the trauma Darlene and my sons suffered through, they never witnessed my sickness and my fear on a daily basis. My siblings never saw the after effects of chemo. I didn't blame them, they had never experienced it, so how could they know about the exhaustion, the diarrhea, the anxiety, the vomiting. the constant worry and fear. We kept this to ourselves. Maybe in retrospect we should've asked for help or at least told them what we were going through. They tried their best, but they weren't with us twenty-four hours seven days a week. They weren't aware how every aspect of life becomes magnified in your mind when dealing with a terminal illness. Before getting sick I most likely would have behaved the same way. They did their best and were there for me, for my colon surgery, the liver surgery and the chemotherapy. I loved them for that, and I appreciate how much they cared for me. I'm sure they were broken hearted and terrified for me and my family.

My brothers and I would on occasion go out for breakfast during my battle with cancer. Other times I would go with my sister Linda. I learned from those get togethers that they did care but they didn't know exactly how to react or what to do or say with what was happening to me. Sometimes you may think that people are insensitive to your needs. Tell them what your feeling so they'll know how to help.

My mother experienced firsthand much of my illness as she lived in the basement apartment of our home. I tried to hide it from her, but she'd hear me throwing up late at night. Hear me walking the floor for hours. She'd phone and ask what was wrong. So as not to worry her I'd say nothing too serious just having trouble sleeping. She spent many days upstairs with us trying to help even though she wasn't well herself. A mother's love is enduring, and I saw in her eyes she suffered for me. I hated putting this burden on her. I always felt especially close to my mother and now even more.

Mid-April is closing in. The appointment with the liver surgeon is looming close and the "normal" fears strike again. The anxiety is becoming intolerable. I can't sleep with so many crazy thoughts rushing in one after the other. I want to run away from my illness, but I can't. I want to stop time, but I can't. I want to speed up time, but I can't. I want to close my eyes and pretend I'm healthy. That it's all been a dream. In my mind I try to go to the sunroom in my cabin. My peaceful place, but I can't. It's overwhelming.

When first diagnosed, I believed death was inevitable. I would put up the good fight but knew deep inside the odds were against me. Sixteen months had passed since that initial diagnosis. I had been septic which should have killed me. I underwent bowel surgery which should have killed me. I suffered two blood clots which should have killed me. My tumors had shrunk. I'd suffered through chemotherapy treatments. I'd had numerous CT scans and waited in small confining rooms to hear the results from oncologists. I'd gone from a death sentence to now having the chance to live. The chance to get my life back. The chance to live my dreams. I now had the hope I'd been searching for since this horrific journey began.

The appointment with the liver surgeon arrives. I suffer a panic attack on the way to the hospital. I've been through hell and back. How much more do I have to endure? How much more does my family have to endure? My continued existence depends on results I'm about to receive. There aren't any words to describe the turmoil raging through your body and mind.

Darlene talks to me in her reassuring tone of voice. "Bob, we've been through so much this past year. I love you and no matter what happens cancer can't take that away." As always, she refuses to think the worst. I sometimes wonder if positive thinking can indeed work miracles.

The surgeon's intern greets us. I immediately think this is a bad omen. Darlene and I hold hands. My heart is racing as the female intern opens the report and reads. "No sign of cancer present on the margins of the portion of the liver that was removed. No sign of cancer in the gallbladder." Weak with relief I hugged Darlene.

The surgeon then came into the room and panic swept over me. Had the intern made a mistake? I'd gone through that once before. A mistake this time would break my spirit. He is very pleased the left side of my liver is cancer free and nicely growing. He said it would take weeks for my liver to grow back to its normal size. Another medical wonder I thought to myself. However, he cautioned I would be watched for the next five years before they can say with certainty that I'm cancer free.

I'm overjoyed. Five years is so much better than six months to live. The surgeon smiles and says, "Tell that lung surgeon to take as good of care of you as I did." I shook his hand and thanked him for saving my life. He smiled once more. "You are too young to die, and we thought let's do everything we can to give him a chance to live." I will forever be grateful to that kind, young, caring surgeon and for his friendship with the lung surgeon. I'm convinced if they hadn't been friends my outcome might have been quite different.

One mountain successfully climbed, it's time to attempt another. My appointment with the lung surgeon is two weeks away. Still, I'm consumed with what's ahead. Sometimes you feel so beat down by everything you've gone through, you become bone weary tired and wish all the fear, worry, procedures, and surgeries would end. Don't get me wrong, I was happy with the liver report, but there are moments when you become overwhelmed. It's like running a twenty-six-mile marathon. Near the end your legs burn. You can hardly breathe. You see the finish line but don't know if you can make it. Your mind and body begs you to stop. Then someone or something motivates you and you cross the finish line. My journey felt like a hundred-mile marathon. I wasn't sure if I'd make it to the finish line.

At times like this Darlene and my boys stepped in with their cheerful outlook inspiring me to continue the fight. How could I quit? How could I give up on them? They travelled this journey with me and deserved my all-out effort. Reaching mile one hundred suddenly didn't seem so far away or so daunting. I continued taking the hash oil. In truth I had no idea if it had been a factor in my success, therefore decided if I stopped taking it my luck would change for the worse. As I've previously stated, I'm not advocating hash oil as a cancer cure but it helped me sleep when burdened with frightening thoughts.

I've no doubt the great doctors, nurses, Darlene, my boys, my siblings, my friends, God, and luck played a key role in my success at this point in the journey. If you don't fight, your loved ones are deprived of the opportunity to fight along with you. Reach out, ask for help. Give those that love you the opportunity to help you. Don't leave them wondering if there was something they could have said or done that would have made a difference. A good friend of the family, a young man, committed suicide and to this day I wonder, did I miss something, is there something I could have done to help him. If only I had noticed, if only he had asked.

7

LUNG SURGERY - IS IT A VIABLE OPTION?

My liver surgery was successful with fantastic results. The end of April 2015 is here and it's time to meet with the lung surgeon. I've beaten all the odds so far. Will this streak of good luck continue?

Darlene and I sit across from the lung surgeon with our hearts in our throats. My insides are quivering as he opened his mouth, and these words flowed out, "Bob, after reviewing your file I believe we may not need to operate." I'm so frantic on the inside I'm paralyzed and can't even utter a word. Darlene speaks up. "What are you saying? We don't understand the meaning of this!" The surgeon explains that the spots on my lungs haven't changed since my first CT scan taken the day Darlene and my sons rushed me to the ER with septicemia. The day my world crumbled.

My voice comes back, and I ask if he's saying the spots aren't cancerous. He can't be certain. If I'm willing, he will delay surgery for six months to see if the spots on my lungs change in any way. My first instinct was to agree, but slowly it dawns on me that perhaps it's the easy way out. Yes, I craved to be finally free to live without further drugs, tests, appointments, and surgery. Then again, I didn't relish the idea of gambling with my life after all I'd been through. I decided to delay any decision on surgery until I discussed it with Darlene, my sons, and more importantly with my oncologist.

I'm constantly expressing my reactions to the news I receive. It's because the journey is like a roller coaster ride. You're frightened, uncertain, fearful, relieved, and even happy at times on this ride you can never see an end to. All you want is to get off and feel safe. The highs and lows can leave you floundering. Darlene and I left the doctor's office amazed, happy, and confused. Had I been given back my life? My sons agreed I needed to speak with the oncologist. If she recommends surgery, I'll go ahead with it.

I call her the next day and explained the results of the liver surgery and the conversation with the lung surgeon. She voiced her surprise and asked for time to review my file. An hour later she called back. "Bob," she said. "I had a deep look into your history. Since the blood clots back in April 2014, we have treated you aggressively. It is my considered opinion you should continue with that approach. I recommend you proceed with the lung surgery."

Even though disappointed to hear this, I knew in my gut that surgery was the right approach. I couldn't just take the easy path. I had to keep fighting. The next morning I called the surgeon and told him what my oncologist had said to me and her advice concerning surgery. He understood and would schedule the surgery for six weeks later, as I needed time to recover from the liver surgery, plus allow time for my liver to attain a normal size. He advises the feasibility of the second lung surgery will depend on the results of the first lung surgery. I'm to call him in six weeks to book the operation.

During these six weeks I try to stay positive and keep busy. When I falter, I take the imaginary trip to the cabin sunroom and watch the spectacular sunset. I'm determined not to second guess my decision to proceed with surgery, though on occasion I'm tempted to cancel. I grow physically stronger each day and the haggard look slowly disappears.

In early May we open up our cabin for the summer. The winter ice has damaged my floating wharf and requires repairs. My brothers Mick, Bill, Ron and Wayne help and soon the wharf is back in the water. I try to encourage my mother to spend the summer weekends with us at the cabin; she refuses as she has never enjoyed the country. Her health is failing and I'm reluctant to leave her alone in her apartment. I talk to my siblings and they agree to look out for her during the weekends while we're at our cabin.

The six-week waiting period is over and Darlene calls to schedule the lung surgery. We find out that the surgeon is booked for the next several weeks which is not ideal. My wife is told to call back in a few days to see if there are any cancellations. She continues to make two or three more calls before my surgery is set. The big date is June 2015.

At this point in my cancer journey I've concluded there are some major keys to survival: gather those you love around you; continue to fight no matter what obstacle is thrown your way; cling to whatever hope your given; stay positive; stay as active as possible and live life as normal as possible. You'll experience good days and plenty of bad ones. You hope and fight for the good days to eventually outnumber the bad days. Before you know it, a positive outlook becomes the norm. Maybe, God willing, I will survive.

It's the day of surgery and the operation is scheduled for eleven a.m. The drive to the hospital is like all the others; the nervous conversation, fear, panic. This time, however, there's one major difference. These emotions are softer, less distressing. The fact that the doctor didn't insist the operation was critical is comforting, instilled hope that I'd receive good news after the surgery.

Darlene and I, along with my mother arrive at the hospital at ten o'clock and check in with the surgical team. We're assigned to the waiting area outside the operating room. Minutes later my sons and siblings arrive. I sit back in my chair and listen to the chatter around me. Everyone is smiling and talking. Though they appear calm I see the worry on their faces. I suddenly have a sense of not being there. My mind is full of worry, full of fear, full of hope, full of anticipation. As the time for surgery approaches I start to shake. My leg bounces up and down. Panic overtakes me. A hand closes over mine and I immediately calm down. It's not my wife's hand; it's my mother's. She tells me not to worry and that I'll be fine. Then she hugs me. At that moment the door opens and the nurse calls my name.

Darlene accompanies me to the pre-op room. I'm handed a complete body anti blood clot mesh outfit to put on. I remove my clothes and struggle into the outfit muttering harsh words as Darlene laughs. She realizes I'm becoming upset. As she helps me I see tears in her eyes. She's been strong throughout my battle. Where would I be without that strength, without her unwavering support? It occurs to me she's just as frightened about the outcome of this surgery as I am. I'll be asleep soon and won't know if I didn't make it. She'll sit in the room with the others waiting, wondering, scared.

It then hits me like a sledgehammer, she's the one who'll

have to deal with my death, help my boys cope. My fears and worries would have ended, hers would last a lifetime. It comforted me to know she'd be there when Josh graduated university, when both boys married and had children of their own. She looks back at me as she is leaving the pre-op room. I'm standing in a white mesh jump suit so tight nothing is left to the imagination. We both laugh. She closes the door behind her and I'm alone!

Transferring from the stretcher to the operating table, I grab the table to help facilitate the move and pull a muscle in my left upper chest. The pain takes my breath away. I didn't tell the nurses for fear the doctor might postpone the operation. The doctor explains what he'll remove during the procedure and what to expect when I wake up in the recovery room. If successful, the second surgery will be scheduled for six weeks time.

Before the anesthetic is administered the surgeon asked me if I'm taking any herbal medicine or anything else he should be aware of. If I mention the hash oil, there's a chance he'll cancel the surgery. I had stopped taking the hash oil two days before the liver surgery and survived. I did the same for the lung surgery. My life is on the line, I take a chance and say no.

Four hours later I wake up in the recovery room with Darlene standing over me beaming the brightest smile I've ever seen. She told me the surgeon came into the waiting room immediately following the operation and told the whole family it went well. He'd removed all five spots and didn't think they were cancerous.

A short while later the surgeon comes in to speak to me and repeated what he'd said to Darlene and all my family. The surgery had gone better than expected. The five spots removed from my right lung didn't look cancerous. One spot appeared different, yet he wasn't concerned. Of course, he couldn't be a hundred percent certain until he had the lab results. The five spots added up to a removal of one third of my lung. He reassured me once my lung healed it would be as before with no breathing problems. If the lab reports show no cancer, there would be no need to operate on my left lung for those spots are identical to those on the right. I thanked him for his great work and the fabulous news he'd given me.

Darlene and I decided in that very moment to take our lives back from this constant cancerous torment. We both felt we had come from death to life. My sons arrived, overjoyed at my prognosis. I told them it looks like they have their father back. I'm going to live. We have the hope we longed for. We'll wait for the lab reports with more optimism than ever before. We talked about our future plans. Yes! I could envision the future as a real possibility and not as a dream or an elusive wish.

Darlene smiled and said we should plan a vacation. What a joy to see her pretty face alight with genuine happiness. For so long she'd forced smiles which never reached her eyes. The suggestion surprised me. Not wanting to dampen her mood or spoil the exhilaration we felt about the news we'd received from the surgeon I agreed. For the first time in eighteen months, I can actually consider a real vacation! I blurted screw cancer. I'm in the mood for living. Darlene booked our tickets to Florida the instant she arrived home.

That night as I lay in bed in the Special Care Unit hooked up to various monitors, so consumed with overwhelming emotions I cried. I had been granted the gift of survival, the gift to dream again, to see and experience the joy of my sons moving ahead with their lives. Not to be stuck in limbo anymore. When you first hear the cancer diagnosis morbid fear is the first emotion. Then denial sets in until finally the acceptance that you are going to die takes hold. Fear, dread, emptiness, panic, anxiety, feeling lost have been my constant companions. The relief makes me giddy. Well, I expect the anesthetic is partly to blame. In a lightning bolt moment another dread wraps around your heart? Did I imagine the good news? I remember my wife's face. Yes. It is true. I have a real shot at a long life.

I'm moved to a ward with three other patients. I'm hooked up to an oxygen and heart monitor and tubes are protruding from my right side. My mother appears and it's obvious she's been crying. She looked tired and happy at the same time. She reaches for my hand and says, "I told you everything would be okay. When you first got sick, I had the feeling that you were going to survive, and you have."

I'm a fifty-eight-year-old man. Yet there's something special about a mother's love that makes you feel like a little boy again who wants his mother to hold him and sooth away all his fears. That he'll be okay. My mother did that for me. My siblings visited for a few minutes overjoyed with my good news. Man, I thought as they left, they really care. I realized how lucky I had been to have such a great support system. I thought about people who suffer alone, those with no support system. How difficult their struggle must be.

I cannot describe the sense of life ebbing inside me that day. It's sad that people, including myself, have to go through a life-threatening experience to truly appreciate the value of life, the value of family, the value of friendships, the value of prayer. We go through each day taking for granted what we have. The idiom "You don't know what you got till it's gone" is so true. You come to appreciate those petty arguments and stupid misunderstandings are irrelevant. They don't matter. Your health, family and friends are what matters, what truly makes life worth living to the fullest. However, the trick is to hold on to that revelation as normalcy returns to your life.

My oxygen levels slowly return to normal. When they do the tube is removed from my right side. It's an uncomfortable procedure as the tube is inside my lung with what the surgeon called reverse stiches. When the tube is pulled out the reverse stiches seal the incision. The surgeon's intern handles the procedure, as with any other profession, they require practice as part of their residency training. He is supervised by the surgeon of course. I'm told to hold my breath as the resident pulls the tube from my chest. I felt the pressure from the moving tube. I'm looking away and don't know it's out. The intern omits to tell me I can breathe again. The surgeon reminds the intern and me that I can carry on breathing again and we all laugh.

I became acquainted with the three other patients on the ward. Two were seriously ill but hadn't given up the fight. The third gentleman was in extremely bad shape. He'd given up and waited to die. How could I blame him? I had no idea the journey he'd traveled with his illness. Maybe he had fought the good fight and the time had finally come for him to rest. Who was I to judge him?

As I looked over at him, I thought perhaps unlike him my fight was finally paying dividends. My will to fight had grown stronger because of my good news. A glimmer of hope can bloom into a fountain of hope. If you're given a timeline of death, don't accept it without a battle. Keep fighting. Find that shred of whatever works for you.

Day five the doctor signs my release papers. He repeats that if the spots removed from my right lung are benign it will be a milestone in my recovery, which means surgery on my left lung won't be necessary. I mention my trip to Florida. I tell him we have the tickets booked and that we are taking a chance that the lab results will be good. I tell the doctor I'm tired of always thinking the worse that now we chose to take the positive out of this and move forward with our lives. He tells me to hold off for at least six weeks, to give myself time to heal. If I fly too soon, the air pressure on the plane could collapse my lung. He hopes my gamble pays off and the tissues samples come back clean from the lab.

Darlene picks me up and both of us comment this is the happiest drive we've taken from the hospital to home in almost two years. Finally, we can see the end of the journey which looks like it may be a good one. The two weeks I have to wait for lab results is hard, yet it's easier this time to be positive.

It's the end of June 2015 and yet again Darlene and I drive to the hospital to see the lung surgeon, to hear the results. Again we're sitting in the small confining room. Again there's that light tap on the door and the doctor enters holding my file. He enquires if I've spoken to my family doctor and received the results? He's surprised when I say no.

My heart pounds as he opens my file. The doctor reads "Spot one, non-cancerous." I have the urge to stop him and ask what this means, but I don't want to interrupt him. I'll ask questions at the end. He continues, "Spot two, non-cancerous; Spot three, non-cancerous; Spot four, non-cancerous." Now for the last spot, the one he was somewhat concerned about. "Spot five, non-cancerous." Darlene and I break down and cry as we hug each other.

We both hug the doctor, and he laughs. He states that too many times he's come into this room to report the opposite news. He further states that it's refreshing and uplifting to deliver the best news anyone will ever hear. His expression reveals how happy he is for us.

I ask him does this mean that the right lung wasn't cancerous. He says that the spots he removed were benign, though there could have been cancer cells in the lung which the chemotherapy destroyed. He adds he couldn't be sure if that was the case. He delivers more good news. As the spots on my left lung are similar to those on my right lung surgery on my left lung is not necessary.

Darlene and I hug the doctor once again. He laughs and says, "Go live your lives." I had my life back. Darlene had her life back; her husband and best friend back. My sons had their father back. My mother had her son back. My siblings had their brother back. My friends had their buddy back.

As we left his office we compare how we felt on the previous walks from the hospital to the way we felt at this moment. We had a full life ahead of us and how we decided to live that life was up to us and not cancer. First thing we did was notify our sons about the good news. My mother came next, and after shedding a few tears said she'd call my siblings. Darlene and I treated ourselves to a celebratory lunch at our favorite restaurant where we made plans for the upcoming Florida vacation. This time we knew the trip would really happen without a care in the world.

8

MY HEART HITS THE FLOOR

It's August 2015 and six weeks had passed since my lung surgery. Myself and Darlene are preparing for our Florida vacation. The idea of a trip still seemed unreal to me. I'm actually going on vacation! A year and a half ago, I thought I would be dead within six months. Now, here I am about to leave for a trip, getting ready to actually enjoy life again. Just me and my wife spending time alone together. Time to enjoy one another's company. Free of dread and uncertainty about the future. Plans, however, can change and often do.

By the time the date of departure arrived two more people have been added to the roster. Josh and Darlene's sister, Val are now coming with us. My wife is excited about the inclusion. How could I refuse after everything she'd been through with me? I agreed on the condition that Josh and Val occupy a separate condo. In truth, I was more than willing to have our youngest son with us. He'd been through the struggle with us and deserved a vacation as well. Bobby was working and couldn't take time off to join us. Val surprised us by paying the extra cost to fly us first class, a thoughtful gesture which I much appreciated.

A few days before the trip my oncologist telephoned with an appointment to see her upon my return. This simple message was a stark reminder that cancer still had its hooks in me. To my astonishment the pending visit to the oncologist never once crossed my mind.

The separate condo units allowed Darlene and I much needed private time. My strength greatly improved as I was able to swim and walk the beach daily. I was somewhat conscious about the scars on my torso during the first walk on the beach. The colon surgery scar ran from the middle of my chest down to my waist. The liver surgery scar ran from my upper chest and around to my right hip. The lung surgery wasn't noticeable as the three incisions were under my right armpit.

Some people stared at the scars and I decided if anyone asked what happened I would reply that I'd been in an accident. The nights are the best in Florida. Walking on the sandy beaches, feeling the warm breeze on your skin, watching people enjoying themselves. Darlene and I were thrilled to have this time together. Time we thought would never happen again. We made up for eighteen months of lost time in three weeks. It felt so good to be alive again. We did the usual 'tourists' activities, taking boat rides, riding the attractions at Disney World, visiting Universal Studio, going to professional baseball games. Darlene and Val shopped every chance they got much to mine and Josh's annoyance.

I'd begun to appreciate life again. Darlene was relaxed. She looked like herself. Life was back in her eyes. I didn't think we would ever be this happy again. The day that all holiday goers dread is at hand, the day to return home. Thoughts of the looming follow-up visit with the oncologist intruded my mind. Worry found me once again. I said nothing and pretended all was well. My family's world shouldn't constantly revolve around me. After all, I'd been extra lucky so far and thrilled to be on a vacation. Josh displayed a look of peace that life was good once more. We deserved this time together.

We're hardly settled back home and its September and time for the appointment with the oncologist. We are in the small waiting room once again and then suddenly the light tap on the door. Knowing the liver and lung surgeries went well I'm not as overpowered with fear and apprehension as on previous occasions. All lab reports were in my favor. I hadn't had a recent CT scan or blood work. No way could the oncologist deliver bad news. No way could she blindside me. I relax. All the angles are covered and I'm safe.

I didn't expect to see my original oncologist, but in she walks having just returned from maternity leave. She says she's happy to see me, yet I perceive a hint of surprise in her eyes. She explains she decided to send my file to the surgical review team even though she felt surgery wasn't an option. Needless to say, she was pleased and astounded to learn I'd undergone the operations. I thanked her for sending my file and expressed my eternal gratitude. I'm convinced, that one decision saved my life. I inquired about her new baby in order to break the tension I felt. She said the delivery went well and her baby was healthy and active, she thanked me for asking.

She's delighted my surgeries were successful and I take this as a signal I won't have to undergo any more medical treatment or procedures. I'm free at last! About to ask what's the next step. She says, "I'll schedule your next round of chemotherapy for the end of September."

My heart hit the floor. Panic swells inside me like a rising tide. I want to run from that tiny room I've grown to hate. I turn to Darlene, her mouth is hung wide open. Her expression scares me. Is she thinking all the hoping and fighting and never giving up will end in defeat? More treatment? More sickness? I'm stunned! I have been blindsided yet again! My insides feel like jelly. I've reached my level of tolerance. I can't go through that nightmare anymore. I'm done! I'm about to tell the doctor no more chemotherapy, that I'll take my chances with whatever happens. I'll live or die with my decision.

The oncologist clues into my unspoken reaction and quickly explains her intent. The operations were indeed a complete success, and she wants to ensure there aren't any rogue cancer cells roaming around inside my body. She expresses her sorrow for the additional chemo treatments, but adds, "Bob, you are a living miracle. I didn't think you would survive. We can't explain why you survived but we're determined to destroy any cancer that may be left."

Darlene calls on her reserves of strength one more time. "Bob, we have been through so much for the past two years. What's another six months? Quitting at this point is the same as drowning a foot from shore." Disappointment and sadness is evident in her voice. Yet she's found the courage, the strength, to travel this final mile to recovery. I can't let her down and refuse the treatment. I grudgingly give my consent to six more chemo rounds. Soon I'd learn that six turned into twelve.

Leaving that confining room I could barely summon the strength to walk up the stairs. I believed the appointment would set me free from cancer's strangling grip. Instead, it had robbed me of the will to fight. As I catch my breath, I'm destroyed that Darlene has to suffer through my treatments again. There's only so much one can take. She's spent her entire life taking care of others. When she was eleven years old her mother was diagnosed with Multiple Sclerosis. From that time on, until Darlene married, she looked after her mother's every need. She cleaned and cooked for the entire household.

When we dated Darlene often couldn't accompany me to events because of her obligations at home. This greatly affected her and caused stress having to bear the brunt of her mother's care. I often wondered why her older sister didn't share any of this responsibility. Darlene by nature is a compassionate person. Perhaps it's a role she easily slipped into.

On our wedding day I made a vow to myself to do whatever was necessary to make Darlene's life better. I promised myself I would never be a burden to her. My goal would be to make her happy, appreciated, and loved. For the past two years I hadn't been able to keep that vow. I let her down. Breaking that promise I made on our wedding day was as difficult to confront as dealing with cancer. Once again my wife would be called upon to care for me. This hurt beyond description.

One moment you're on top of the world, the next you're down in the dirt. It's an unbelievable challenge to drag yourself up but you must. You dust yourself off and continue the fight. If you're going through cancer, a mental illness or any other situation that causes you to question your very existence, don't give up. Fight on. I know it's easier said than done. Many times I wanted to give up. I believed I can't do this anymore. The ever-present fear, torment and anxiety beats you down. If only it would subside, leave me in peace. Please let it all end, one way or another.

On several occasions during my cancer journey I stood on the edge of the wharf at my cabin contemplating ending it all. Let myself fall in and drift away. Let all the torment evaporate. If I jump in the peace I've searched for, craved for, wished for, with all my being would flow through me. Thank God I remained on the wharf. Images of Darlene and my boys would flash inside my head. What sort of message would I send them by ending it all? Reality can't be brushed aside. There are times when the struggle beats you down and you can't bring yourself to consider your loved ones during those desperate episodes, but you must.

That's the precise moment you have to stop and reflect on how your decision would affect your loved ones. Their torment would only increase, saddled with a burden they'll never forget, one not of their own making. They'll be forever plagued with doubt. Could they have done more to help you? Did they miss a plea for help from you? As often happens, the blame for your death will shift to them. I could never place that burden on the family I loved.

When you reach what you feel is the lowest point of your life lean on your loved ones and your support systems. Reach out for help. What a wonderful message this gives your loved ones. You care enough about them to live for yourself and for them. Years ago I once asked my nephew, Michael to sing Louis Armstrong's song "What a Wonderfull World" at my gravesite. Since the onset of my illness living had become a monumental challenge and now the song had little meaning for me. Give life a chance. It can improve even though you feel trapped in a thick fog and can't see beyond the illness. If you find yourself standing on the edge of the wharf, please don't jump. Things can get better. Lately the words from that song bring me joy once more. And perhaps I'll ask my nephew to sing once again that beautiful song at my gravesite, years from now.

I begin the new round of chemo in September 2015.

Round thirteen to date. Round one of the second set. My siblings have expressed they're upbeat about the treatments which will hunt down and kill every rogue cancer cell. They tell me that once and for all I'll be free, healthy, and alive. This time they're not pretending all will be well. It's obvious by their enthusiasm they mean what they say. Their positivity begins to rub off.

My port hasn't been removed so that's one less procedure to endure. I greet the same wonderful nurses in the unit eagerly helping all those scared people. Being an old hand at this, I'm not as distraught as I was that very first treatment. Experience can be a great reliever. I'm prepared for the long hours waiting for my drugs to be mixed. Sitting for hours as the toxic mixture is pumped inside you, then taking home the bottle attached to your chest for three days. The steroids taken for three days followed by sickness. You feel better on day eleven only to return to the clinic on day fourteen for a repeat of the punishment. It sucks. However, the hope it's killing whatever remnants of cancer lurking in you burns bright.

The first six treatments of this new round caused no major setbacks apart from the usual sickness and loss of taste. Things changed with round seven. My white blood cell count was low, and the chemo had to be delayed for several hours until the count returns to a level that can tolerate the toxic drugs without causing me problems. A few days later at home I experienced numbness in my feet and fingertips. I'd been warned that was a possible side effect from a specific drug used to kill small cancer cells. My oncologist warned me to let her know immediately about any different adverse effects. Upon advising her she promptly took me off the drug as she felt I'd received enough of the drug to do the job and therefore didn't want to cause any further damage to my toes and fingers.

The numbness and pain in my feet and fingers is permanent. It's a constant reminder of my battle with cancer. I consider it a small price to pay for the luxury of living a long, pretty much healthy life. This affliction does have its drawbacks. I was an avid jogger. When I run the pain in my feet is unbearable. The oncologist asked what was the one thing I could do pre cancer but unable to do post cancer. My immediate response was running. Running kept me fit both physically and mentally. My son, Josh makes it a point to tell me there's other means to stay fit. Someday I'll take his advice and get back to exercising.

An old friend from work once said exercising is like money in the bank when it comes to your health. It's there when you need it. I've withdrawn all my exercise currency fighting cancer. I need to get active and start replenishing my exercise bank account.

In the beginning, January 2014, when I was taking my very first chemotherapy treatment, I heard a bell ring outside the cancer clinic. The nurse explained that it signified someone had completed their last round of chemo and were hopefully cancer free. I thought, here I am round one I doubted I'd ever get the opportunity to ring the bell. Here I am hooked up to toxic drugs, scared and waiting for the cancer to kill me. I was always in good physical shape now I'm sitting here waiting to die. I'm never going to be granted the privilege of ringing that damn bell. Darlene sat next to me and I wondered did the same thought cross her mind.

Two years ago I'd been given six months to live. Miraculously, two years later I'm still alive and trudging through my last rounds of chemo. I thought you better believe I'm going to ring that bell. I'm living proof you never give up; you always cling to whatever bit of hope is flung your way. I'm elated with the idea that very soon I'll ring that bell with my whole family in attendance.

My final round of chemo, round twenty four, finished the end of January, 2016. I had a CT scan and was scheduled to meet with my oncologist in early February. I'd come to detest the small room and the light tap on the door. The oncologist reports the scan didn't show any sign of cancer. She'd never come right out and say I was cancer free. It irked me that she always held back. I understand they have to be cautious and not raise spirits when not one hundred percent positive. You must wait those magical five years before the words "cancer free" are spoken. She couldn't, wouldn't, breach that medical code. I would be undergoing CT scans every six months for the next three years. From the moment we left the doctor's office that day I planned on moving forward with my life in the belief I was indeed cancer free.

I rang the bell on February 15, 2016, a little over two years since my initial diagnosis. My death sentence had been commuted and I'd been set free. Darlene and I invited all those who had helped me travel my journey. We gathered in the lobby of the clinic where the bell is situated. As Darlene, Josh, Bobby and my mother stood by my side I glanced over the crowd to make sure no one was missing. I couldn't see my brother, Wayne who'd been instrumental in my fight. There was no way I'd ring the bell without him. He arrived twenty minutes later with his wife. She'd come from a doctor's appointment of her own. All those I loved and cared for were present. I was ready to ring the bell of life! The bell of hope!

As I reached up my arm to pull the string, I thought about all I'd gone through; the cancer news, the chemotherapy, the blood clots, the good news the tumors had shrunk, the anxiety worrying and waiting for tests results, wondering if surgery was possible, then waiting for more biopsy results and the almost debilitating disappointment learning about a second round of chemotherapy. How could I forget that small, suffocating room and the light tap on the door. Pure fear had dogged my every waking hour. Now I felt weightless from its departure.

It was a journey I'd never imagined taking. Yet here I am about to end this journey by ringing the bell of hope. The bell of life. I thought about the patients at this very moment in the cancer clinic suffering through chemo treatments. Hearing the bell ring. I know exactly what they are thinking and feeling. One arm around Darlene I rang the bell with tears in my eyes. My family applauded.

The sound of the bell made me feel like Clarence the angel in the Christmas classic film "It's a Wonderful Life" with Jimmy Stewart. Clarence is finally awarded his wings for performing a good deed. I had gotten my wings of life back. It may sound silly, but my spirit had returned as well. I seemed to soar above the crowd looking down at each and every one. Seeing their smiles, their joy, and their relief. Wayne, the big, strong fireman had tears in his eyes. Throughout my journey I often called on my deceased father Ron and my deceased sister Joan to watch over me. To protect me. I hold their pictures in my hand and thanked them for I know they were in some way responsible for my newfound health.

It's at these moments you realize the importance of family and friends in your life. The trick is to never forget that sentiment. Ringing the bell was one of the major milestones in my cancer journey. Despite several more paces left to travel in the journey, I left the cancer clinic re-energized.

We invited family and friends to our home for a celebratory lunch.

For the next two months my goal is to forget about cancer and the upcoming scan in April. I'm feeling so good Darlene books another trip to Florida. I preferred another destination but gave in since I loved how relaxed and at ease she felt there.

I caught a bad flu in mid-March and quickly recovered. Soon after I had the regular blood work and CT scan. Then the waiting room and the tap on the door and an intern enters. I freeze for I haven't had much luck with interns. My blood work is fine. Her expression warns me the hammer is about to crash down on my head. The CT scan has shown a spot on my right lung. Intense fear rushed over me. In an instant my life is turned upside down once again. The radiologist isn't sure whether or not the spot is cancerous. I ask if surgery is an option. Shockingly she responds with utter sarcasm, "We can't remove everything." I'd been through hell and didn't appreciate her callous reply and I told her so.

Once that awkward moment had passed, I mention my recent flu. She was surprised to hear that and suggested the spot on my lung could be left over infection from the congestion. The intern scheduled another CT scan for September 2016. How many more times do I have to leave the clinic devastated? How many more setbacks for me and my family? I chose to focus on the possibility the spot was indeed left-over infection. If the cancer has returned, I'll grit my teeth and enter the battle again.

The Florida trip was set for June 2016. How could I go with peace of mind that perhaps cancer had reared its ugly head again? How could we enjoy the trip? I wanted to cancel. Darlene suggested we take the time while in Florida to relax and not think about cancer. Worrying or staying home wouldn't help. A change of scenery might bring about a change of mind. The month and a half before we leave for the trip is difficult for me. It helps that I'm feeling healthy and energetic which I take as a good sign that perhaps the spot on my lung is actually left-over infection from the flu. I was proud to be able to think this way for at least seventy percent of the time. As June 8th is approaching Darlene and I are truly excited about the trip.

9

ALL CONSUMING GUILT

June 1, 2016 Wayne drops by my home to see how I'm doing. We chat about my upcoming trip to Florida and about his daughters and his grandchildren with whom he's close. I can tell he's worried about something although it's obvious he doesn't want to burden me with his troubles. I think maybe I can finally help him in some small way. I asked how everything was with him and his family. He's reluctant at first to say anything but eventually explains his wife isn't well. She is in kidney failure and has to go on dialysis. He's concerned and upset, even becoming emotional as he tells the story.

I tried to offer him hope that everything would be okay. The same hope I'd always sought. I could tell those words didn't seem to help him. We talked a little more about his grandchildren and how they were doing in school. Darlene and I stood at the window watching him walk to his car. We both commented he didn't look well. We understood he was worried about his wife, yet it went further than that. He looked tired, haggard, not his usual robust healthy appearance.

Several days later on his daily visit to my mother for tea and toast he was struck with a sudden case of nausea and a severe pain in his middle back. He leaves immediately without finishing his breakfast which was absolutely out of the norm for him. My mother calls his house to see how he is doing and he tells her he's okay. She hears the strain in his voice and wants to go to his home to see for herself that he's fine. Meanwhile his pain worsens, and he can't stop vomiting. His wife and daughter rush him to the hospital where he's diagnosed with acute pancreatitis. He's left for the hospital by the time our mother reached his house.

In order to survive you have to fight but you also have to be lucky. I was lucky I ended up with some fantastic doctors who helped save my life. My brother on the other hand wasn't so lucky. His doctor was uncaring, to say it nicely, he was useless. He made assumptions about my brother and I believe based his course of treatment on those assumptions. Had he started my brother on the proper treatment plan for pancreatitis he would have had a chance to fight like I was given. He wasn't treated with the dignity or respect he deserved.

I visited Wayne in the hospital the day before I was due to leave for Florida. The big strong brother I knew now looked physically weak. I felt so sad for him. Some of his color had returned though he looked in distress. I asked him when he expected to go home. He wasn't himself and it made me nervous. I told him I'd postpone my trip until he was well. He insisted I not cancel as he would be released in a few days. He said "you've suffered enough and you deserve a holiday. I'll be fine. You go and enjoy yourself." Even at this low point in his life he was more concerned for me. As I was leaving, I whispered in his ear, "You always told me to stay strong and fight, will you promise to do the same?" He looked up at me and said, "You know I will."

I decided that night to go ahead with my plans. Was it a selfish move? I don't know the answer. However, the decision haunts me to this day. I lost three precious weeks with my brother. I knew the health care system well. Perhaps I could have done something to help him. In reality what could I possibly do? Just being there for him maybe could have helped in some small way. His wife and daughters demanded the best care for him which he never received until it was too late. I'll never forgive myself for letting him down. Should I have cancelled our trip? I struggle with the answer to that question every day.

At five a.m. on June 8th Darlene and I board the plane. As it taxis down the runway for takeoff I'm happy yet disturbed. Have I done the right thing by leaving my brother? The spot on my lung is ever present in my thoughts. Darlene is sitting beside me, terrified of flying but willing to brave it for a few weeks of relaxation. I know I have to put aside all negativity, or the trip will be ruined for her. Sometimes you have to think of others, it's not always about you and your feelings.

We arrive in Tampa at one p.m. Wayne is constantly on my mind. I keep it from Darlene. I think maybe we should have cancelled our trip. Darlene would have been OK if we had. The decision was on me.

The first two weeks are relaxing and I'm enjoying this time with my wife. The sun filled days refresh us. Walking on the beach watching the sun set is rejuvenating. We visited Disney World and sat on the same bench as we had done on our honeymoon in May 1982. We recall the playful argument we had that day concerning which direction to go to enter the park. Darlene chose left. I chose right. She won the argument and we turned left. This time we sit on the same bench as we enter the park, we have the same playful argument, this time we turn right.

We visited Disney Springs on June 11, 2016; apparently the same day the Pulse Night club shooter had been there contemplating whether to attack Disney Springs or the Club. The next night June 12th, 2016 he attacked the Pulse Night Club killing forty nine and wounding fifty three. Such a sad and tragic waste of human life. I was fighting for my life; Wayne was fighting for his. Yet some crazy lunatic can buy a gun and destroy forty nine lives, forty nine families in just minutes.

During our marriage I occasionally seranaded Darlene with the song "Do you like Pina Colada" by Rupert Homes. It tells the story of a man who feels his relationship with his wife has lost its excitement. He puts an advertisement in the paper listing activities he'd like a partner to enjoy. He receives a response from a woman who enjoys the same things as him. She turns out to be his wife. We always make it a priority to maintain love and excitement in our relationship. However, if you become complacent and take the relationship for granted you lose your connection. When I'd sense this emotional separation, I'd sing the song as a reminder. Darlene would receive the message every time. There was no reason to sing that song during this trip.

While in Florida, the topic of cancer, illness and the coming CT scan were off limits. Wayne was right to insist Darlene and I needed special time alone. I still wonder if perhaps he needed me more. The vacation is drawing to an end. I'll have to confront the possibility I have lung cancer.

While on vacation I phoned Wayne a number of times to check on him. His wife would always answer and immediately pass the phone to him. He'd say he was fine and hand the phone back to her. She'd confirm that he was okay. I knew that wasn't true. Wayne was a talker, a joker. Now he barely uttered a word. I called my mother who repeated that Wayne was fine. A mother can never disguise the anguish and concern for her child. It resounded in her voice. I could tell something was wrong.

The last day of our vacation we drive along the beach with the sun in the rear-view mirror. It's thirty degrees Celsius and the beach is lined with people enjoying the pleasant weather. The trip has been great, however getting home to see how my brother is doing is my number one concern right now.

Reality sets in. I have to go home. My brother needs me. The flight gets in late at night and immediately worry sets in with a vengeance. I may have lung cancer and my brother is ill. I need to find out for myself how he is doing. I have to stay focused forget my worries and concentrate on my brother.

Josh picks us up at the airport and I enquire how Uncle Wayne is doing. He's silent for a moment. "Dad, he is not good. He's been in the hospital for a week. He wanted the truth kept from you and mom while you were in Florida."

Everyone kept it from me until I returned from my vacation, that was my brother's request. Wayne was struggling for life yet was concerned for my happiness. The doctors have no idea what's happening to him. Darlene and I head straight for the hospital. My big, strong, independent brother is being fed by his wife. He looks extremely weak, down, withdrawn and has lost weight. I managed not to breakdown for I have to stay strong for him just as he had for me. He'd layed in bed at home for fifteen days with no medication prescribed being told that time would heal his pancreas.

Outside the hospital room I ask his wife what happened. She says he grew worse day by day and she had no choice but to take him to the hospital. The doctors diagnosed him with acute pancreatitis. I'm confused for this was the original diagnosis. I still blame the doctor who first saw him all those weeks ago for the deterioration of my brother's condition. Fury and anger accost me, but I hold back. This isn't the time to vent.

Anger has replaced any worry I felt for myself and I ask Wayne's wife how I can help. She's close to tears and asks me to pray for his recovery. It's in God's hands now. We return to his room, and he enquires how my vacation went. I'm more concerned for him and ask how he's feeling. He gives the same answer he's given every time he's asked. "I'm doing fine."

I'm so glad I visited him that night for the next day he took a dramatic turn for the worse. Doctors are in his room when Darlene and I arrive. All visitors are asked to leave. Alarms are going off and more doctors rush into his room. I try to go to my brother, but I'm prevented by the doctors. His wife and daughters are in the corridor crying. All our siblings arrive and are bewildered. What's going on? What's happening, this big strong man is now fighting for his life. I felt so useless, so sad, and so desperate; there was nothing I could do to help him. I missed three weeks that I was on vacation. Three weeks that I could have spent with him. Last night could be the last time I ever get to speak with him. I was devastated. Maybe if I had stayed home and hadn't gone on vacation I could have done something. These are the questions to which I'll never get the answer.

Life doesn't standstill because you are fighting a life-threatening illness. I'm stunned my brother is fighting for his life. I'm worried about him but also worried about myself. I'm feeling guilty for going on vacation and leaving him. I'm praying for him. I'm overwhelmed. Fear and depression take root. Wayne is fighting for his life, and I have to undergo another CT scan. I can't go to the cabin and sit in the sunroom to calm myself. Wayne's life is in the balance, looking at him I realize he is in serious trouble.

I hear gasps. My sisters are all crying. Wayne's lying motionless, his eyes closed as several doctors are pushing his bed towards the elevator. He's transferred to the Intensive Care Unit where he's put into an induced coma and put on a ventilator. When I see him hooked up to monitors and unresponsive my legs almost fall out from beneath me. He's helpless. We can't talk to him. I want to take him in my arms and reassure him everything will be okay. The stark reality settles in my soul. He's in deep trouble. His wife and daughters are distraught. If only I could tell them he'll pull through. My brother hasn't been afforded that chance to fight to live. His survival is now truly in God's hands, and his doctors.

Guilt claws at my heart and forces me from the ICU. Why wasn't Wayne given a chance to fight as I had been? Do his daughters have the same thoughts? No matter your strength there will be times you'll feel defeat. The fight will seem to have deserted you. This was one of those times for me. You have no choice but to battle through the down times. I know my brother would want me to be strong and I decide if my cancer is back, I will fight it. Wayne isn't in a position to fight. I can and I will not die. My brother's chance to fight has been stolen from him. I'll honor him by working that much harder to achieve a long, fulfilling life, he would want that.

Wayne's condition steadily deteriorates thus overriding my worry about my impending CT scan. Darlene and I visit him every night. We hold his hand and pray we'll be lucky enough to be granted another miracle. He's woken from the induced coma and is confused at first. His hands are strapped to the railings of the bed to prevent him from pulling out his numerous tubes. I smother at the sight. He doesn't communicate at all, he just lies there and stares straight ahead. We are terrified maybe he has had a stroke. I hope he is okay and he is gone to that imaginary place he told me to go to when I was scared.

He couldn't get up and fight. He's strapped to the bed like a prisoner. He couldn't go for a walk with his daughters who are the light of his world. He couldn't go for drives. I wonder if he had accepted death. He wasn't given another choice. I feel terribly guilty. I was lost. A tracheotomy is inserted to help him breathe. He's rushed to surgery to repair his pancreas. It's so damaged the surgeon said it was softer than tissue paper. He's now hooked up to even more machines. He is placed on life support. I saw the emptiness in his eyes. Our mother refuses to leave him although she is unwell.

Wayne's daughters often commented on how much I remind them of their father. Though they didn't realize it, this made me feel even more guilty. I'm alive and their father is close to death. It was beyond my power to give him the strength he needed to fight, as he had done for me. He was cheated the way I hadn't been and that gave me courage to carry on for his sake. I felt guilty about this. I could fight to live their father wasn't given that chance. Knowing him I'm sure he would have fought to survive and he would have wanted me to continue my fight.

By July 30th Wayne has been in ICU three weeks. The doctor summons his wife, children and siblings to the ICU waiting room for a meeting to discuss his lack of progress.

Everything medically possible has been done for him. It's time to make that dreadful decision no one ever wants to face. Removal from life support is advised. Once this happens, he'll pass away within an hour or two. His wife and daughters break down. This is a living nightmare, and it takes several minutes before they internalize what's been asked of them. They come to terms with the knowledge they had to let him go and give their consent. He's suffered enough and deserved peace.

My brother tried his best to support me when I was told I had six months to live. He did his best to help me, now here I am still alive while he will most likely die in a few hours. I didn't know what to say or do. I felt this immense sense of loneliness. Wayne's untimely and unnecessary death has left a deep scar in my heart.

Each of us visits him for one last time to say good-bye, to wish him a safe journey into the hands of our father and sister. I held his hand and told him I was sorry: that I would miss him. I thanked him for caring about me when I needed his support the most. Then I said good-bye to my brother, the big, strong fireman. That's how I'll remember him. Not the frail thin man I was looking down at.

2:00 am on July 31st, 2016, Wayne took his last breath. He was four days from his 63rd birthday. Our mother lost our father, her husband Ron, when he was fifty-six, she was fifty years old at the time. She lost our sister, her daughter, Joan who was fifty-eight. Now her son Wayne was gone at a young age. I was nearly sixty at the time and had been fighting cancer for almost three years. I swore that day my mother was not going to see another son die.

Wayne's funeral took place on an overcast, unusually cool day in August. To add more tragedy, it was his youngest daughter's birthday. The very life seemed to have gone out of my mother and we feared she might collapse. She was stronger than we gave her credit for, and she made it through. Most people rise to the occasion when faced with hardship. We are stronger than we believe we are.

In the aftermath of the funeral my will to fight had been severely diminished. Grief takes a toll on healthy, happy people. I had to fight through grief over my brother's death. Fight against the guilt I'd let him down. My spirit is shattered, and I sink into a deep depression. My brother's bravery and words of encouragement cut through my anguish and mental fatigue. His memory built me up once more. If the spot on my right lung was cancerous, I'd suffer through another surgery and more chemotherapy if required. My respect and love for Wayne guided me back into reality and the will to continue the fight.

10

LIFE MUST GO ON

The remainder of August 2016 is warm and sunny and we spend most of the weekends at our cabin. The drive along the open highway with nothing but trees and greenery on each side instills in me a sense of peace. I try to stay busy at the cabin seeking out little jobs. I take the boat for a spin on the lake. Wayne's death never leaves my mind. Grief and loss is written all over his wife and two daughters faces. It's as if part of them has been stolen away.

I have to stay positive. I've never broken a promise to my mother, and I can't break my silent promise that another son wouldn't die. I hold all my fears inside. Truly, I'm sick of them dogging my every thought, day after day, like an itch I can't scratch. My family has listened to them over and over for years and must be just as tired of hearing them as I am of repeating them.

September 2016, the day for my CT scan and blood work has been a long time coming. Yet again, the waiting game commences. I'm due to meet with the oncologist a week following the tests. This three-year routine I've struggled through weighs me down. I'm fed up and wish it was all over. Today I realize grief for my brother was partly responsible for my agitation. Surprisingly the week after the CT scan goes by quickly. Darlene and I are seated in that small room waiting for that light tap on the door. It opens and the oncologist walks in without having tapped as she always does. I was so startled by this my mouth actually gaped open. Lord! What disastrous news does she have for me! Why do we always anticipate the worst? I've come to believe it's a defense mechanism to prepare us.

The oncologist is aware how stressed we've become waiting for results. She's barely inside the room when she opens her mouth to speak. My heart is pounding. My leg is bouncing up and down. My insides are numb and I'm quivering all over. I hear her voice, yet it sounds like a faraway echo. I can't seem to focus in on the words. "The CT scan is perfect."

My brain snaps to attention as the oncologist continues to speak. "The spot on your lung is gone. It must have been left over infection from your flu. Your blood work is also perfect."

She's just given me a clean bill of health. I want to shout for joy. Most of all I want to get out of that miniature room. My wife has a load of questions. Will there be more chemotherapy? When is the next CT scan? The next blood test. I'm itching to run out of there and don't hear one single answer. I want to celebrate life. I finally cue in that Darlene is thanking the doctor. She's happy for us and wishes us both good luck. I thank her and fly out the door.

I sprint up the stairs eager to get out of the Cancer Clinic. The same stairs on which many times before I didn't have the strength to climb. I run to the car not even waiting for Darlene. She reaches me minutes later. "Bob," she cries.

"No more chemotherapy. The cancer is gone. We're finally free of this torment." She breaks the news that another CT scan and blood work is scheduled for six months's time.

This brings me down a little, but I have to hold on to the fact I was just given back my life. So, I say what the hell. I'm not going to worry about tests that are so far in the future. I'll worry later; month six is time enough to worry. Three years ago all I had left to live was six months, now I think six months is a life time. I phoned my sons and mother. She cries at the good news and her voice sounds full of energy. I didn't realize until that moment how much I missed that. She is anxious to hang up so she can call the rest of her children and spread the news. I imagine their reactions. They've walked with me on that road froth with cancer. It's high time we all get off it.

It takes a few days to assimilate the news the oncologist has given me. It looks like I'm finally free of the trappings of cancer. I'm cured! These two words are the greatest and most meaningful I will ever hear. I'm determined to use the next months to enjoy all the good things life has to offer. I can look forward to Christmas and Easter without worrying about cancer. I feel like a hundred-pound boulder which has been strapped to my shoulders for three and a half agonizing grueling years has been lifted off and I can straighten up with ease. At first this is an odd sensation. The boulder had become a constant companion. Now it's gone and you feel light enough to float. It will take time to adjust to this new freedom.

Darlene looks relaxed and can't stop smiling. And in that smile, I know the fight was worth it, even though your body begs you to let go, to let the struggle go. When you're in the full throes of fighting to survive it's impossible to envision the future. All plans are thrown out the door. All you are guaranteed is the present. You don't know if you'll be alive to push on another day, week, or month. Everything revolves around "now'." The moment, I, my family, my mother, siblings, and friends have prayed for is here. The future is mine. What a sense of peace, a sense of life swells within me!

I have been dealing with cancer for eleven years beginning with the prostrate in 2006. This Christmas will be the best since 2005. Back then I lived life to the fullest. I wanted to relive those carefree days. Before a life-threatening illness, I don't believe we really appreciate what we have in terms of our health or the people who love us. We tend to take life for granted. Count your blessings when waking up next to a spouse or partner, attending a child's baseball or hockey game, meeting with friends for a drink or a meal. Take the time to really enjoy a sunset, so what if it rains and an event is cancelled. So what if you spend two hundred dollars for a meal. When you wake in the morning appreciate the fact you woke up. Appreciate seeing your child graduate from university, seeing that child marry. Growing old with loved ones around you. Forgive those who've harmed you in some way.

When cancer storms into your life, you discover what is really important and weed out the trivial things. I'm convinced that people who are sincerely happy and content have figured this out before any traumatic illness or event comes their way. Darlene, perhaps from her own life experience growing up is one of those lucky people. My goal is to appreciate and never revert to the old ways of complacency. I never want to forget the true value of life. Now healthy once more I pray that I'll keep everything in proper perspective.

This Christmas would be festive with the house decorated once again. I'd open my gifts on Christmas day, relish the turkey dinner and welcome friends and family. The Christmas spirit of love and goodwill will abound in my home. Always love, respect and treat others with dignity. Never take anyone or anything for granted. Always remember the importance of the "small stuff." It's sad a serious illness was the catalyst to making me appreciate what I had. Material things are replaceable. The love of my wife, my sons, my mother, my siblings, and my friends are precious and irreplaceable.

I now truly understood the importance of taking time to really listen, to help in any way possible. Never ridicule or cast aside another's feelings. Never tell them in a flippant tone to "get over" whatever phobia or fear they have. Don't make them feel inadequate. Don't make them feel they can't confide in you. I've always tried to be a caring person but now I have learned a little understanding and empathy can help in ways you'll never know.

In March 2017 I have another CT scan and blood work done. A week later Darlene and I are once again in the small room. I won't say I wasn't worried, but the fact I felt healthy lessened the anxiety. This time the oncologist tapped before entering and immediately said, even before sitting down, "Bob, everything is great, no sign of cancer, see you in September." I'd been granted another six months to enjoy the little things in life, a lesson I would never forget.

I would have moments when the dread and fear returned, however Darlene would remind me to get back to living, to appreciating life. I float out of the room and once again run up the stairs which have become a symbol of my renewed good health. I phone my family with the news. I wish I could talk to my brother, Wayne and tell him the good news.

We go to his grave, unaware at the time his wife will pass in June, a mere ten months after his death. I talk to him as if he's there with me, listening. I believe he shed another tear for me that day. This time it's a tear of happiness. He'd given me strength, showed up when I needed his advice. I believed I hadn't done that for him. I'd put myself first and gone on that God blessed Florida trip. To this day I can't forgive myself for missing those last few precious weeks with him. I miss my brother. I miss his guidance.

Guilt wears you down both mentally and physically. I suspect Wayne knew his illness would take him, yet his concern for me never wavered. He knew I needed that Florida vacation, and the fact he wouldn't allow family to tell me his health was waning while I was away should free me from guilt. Knowing something still doesn't take away the regret or the guilt.

We take another holiday in May of 2017. We hop in the car and see where it takes us. I have an idea that Darlene has a specific destination in mind though she insists she doesn't. I always wanted to see Houston, New Orleans, and Los Angeles. It's raining when we leave which doesn't dampen our mood. Two days later we arrive in Bangor, Maine on a sunny warm day. We leave the next morning for Cape Cod as the Kennedy family has always fascinated Darlene. We walk the beach and converse with the locals who are friendly and welcoming. They recount the history of Cape Cod as well as the Kennedy's time in residence.

After Cape Cod Darlene suggests we drive to Savannah, Georgia, arriving late at night we seek out a hotel, spending the next day touring the city. We'd stopped off there once before on our way to Florida which reinforces the notion she had a plan as to where she wanted to go from the start. As we lay in bed that night, I asked her for a suggestion about our next destination. She replies as if the idea has just occurred to her that Dave and Joanne, friends who live in our neighborhood, are staying at their condo in Florida. We should visit them.

I laugh and say isn't it a coincidence we end up in Savannah only one day's drive from Florida. My preference was Houston then down to New Orleans. I give in. It felt good to do something just for Darlene after she'd put her life on hold for me. It's refreshing and wondrous not dwelling on cancer, not dwelling on death. What a shift in circumstances! My biggest concern is deciding on New Orleans or Florida. The next morning we head to Florida. As we're driving, I play the Eagles CD and sing along, Darlene joins in. Something she'd never done before. This is great, I thought. She's really and truly happy for the first time in years. I love my wife, my eyes swell with tears thinking how great life is. There's no need to sing Pina Colada this day.

Life is perfect. I never expected it was possible to feel this free and at peace. I recall the time I stood on the wharf at the cabin contemplating ending my life. I'd miss this time with Darlene. When you've sunk to the lowest point of your life you have to somehow find a way to rise above the depression. Think about those you'd leave behind. As I sat next to my wife the fight, the journey, the pain, and the torment was worth it. There were many times I wanted to give up. My loved ones wouldn't let me. God bless them for standing by me, for staying strong when I couldn't.

We rent a condo in Florida and for two weeks walk the beach, enjoy the sunsets, enjoy the soothing sound of waves washing onto the shore from the bedroom. Make love free of worries and doubt. We spend time with Dave and Joanne. They're an easy-going couple and fun to be around. There's no pressure, no stress. Simply a husband-and-wife spending time with good friends. We swim, soak up the sun and enjoy their company. Cancer and sickness is never discussed. I drink a few cold beers with Dave by the pool side in one-hundred-degree heat.

Dave and Joanne invite us to stay an extra week with them in their condo. We declined as we'd been away from home for three weeks. Darlene was missing our sons.

The next day we leave to begin the five day drive home. An hour away from home we stop at a restaurant for a meal, for the simple reason neither of us were quite ready to end the vacation. As we got back into the car all the fears and anxiety over the last three and a half years bombarded me. The urge to turn the car around and head west was almost overpowering. As sudden as these emotions swept over me, they vanished and we headed east, towards home.

11

***

I MADE THE RIGHT DECISION!

My sons and my mother greet us as we come through the front door of our home. Darlene and I talk about the trip and hand out the gifts we brought back for each of them. I noticed my mother was quiet, distant. There was an emptiness in her eyes that pained me. My brother's death had taken something from her. At times she seemed confused, disoriented. She was eighty-eight years old and I was afraid death was coming for her. My mother's health had been declining since my cancer diagnosis. I hoped I wasn't the reason.

We spend most weekends during that summer at our cabin as usual. Repeated requests for our mother to join us failed. She didn't enjoy cabin life. September rolled around bringing with it my CT scan and blood work along with the usual fear and anxiety waiting for the results. All went extremely well. The oncologist, always professional and over cautious in her reports, in my opinion at least, finally expressed her delight and amazement. I had survived! My family doctor called me the "miracle man." No medical professional could explain why I survived. For the next three years I routinely have CT scans and blood work which all come back with no sign of cancer.

I had been battling cancer struggling to live for the past four years. I had received the news for which I had been hoping for, praying for. Finally, it appeared I was going to live. My mother had been by my side for this long four year battle. She deserved to understand and appreciate this good news. It broke my heart, my mother was aging and her life was coming to an end. I felt relieved for my situation but yet devastated for what my mother was going through. Periods of forgetfulness and confusion were beginning to take its toll on her.

My relationship with my mother was an important part of my life. She instilled in me many of the qualities I drew upon to survive. Her declining health affected me as I watched her loose her battle for survival. She loved life and had given that love of life to me. My mother was fading away while I was fighting to live.

For fifty-three of my now sixty-seven years of life I lived with my mother. The first twenty-six I lived in her home, and for twenty-seven years she lived in my home. I truly miss her, my sons miss our Sunday dinners together. She was a big part of their lives for twenty-seven years. My mother was naturally a happy pleasant woman. Josh, my youngest son was one month old when she moved into our basement apartment. She'd tell him she had a special love for him, but he had to promise not to tell anyone. My mother joined us for the boys birthdays, and also mine and Darlene's. She joined us for drives, ate Sunday dinner with us, and accompanied us on vacations. She was an everyday part of our life. She was a part of our family. We called her the "Boss" as she let us know her feelings on the proper way to raise our sons. My mother and I often joked that Darlene was the boss in training.

I'd fought cancer during the years our mother's health declined. She required more and more care and support. Darlene and I were there twenty-four hours, seven days a week. We were in constant communication with the home care workers, and we were often called down to the apartment to help because my mother's mobility had become an issue. Most of my siblings didn't grasp the level of stress and pressure we felt, wondering if she had fallen during the night or if she'd had a stroke or heart attack. The further removed you are from a situation, the easier it is to put it from your mind. The toilet flushing late at night signaled she was alive much to our relief.

I believe my siblings, with a few exceptions never understood the stress and anxiety we were going through. Trying to survive myself, while wanting our mother to remain in the apartment where she felt safe and loved. Some family members wanted to put her in a home. In truth, those who sided for the home were right, realizing it would be wiser and kinder for her to be in a place where she'd receive the twenty-four hour care she needed. It was truly suggested out of love for her.

Sadly my mother's health continued to deteriorate. Several times she was hospitalized with congestive heart failure. Other times for serious bladder infections and pneumonia. My brother's death haunted my mother; she'd often refer to him as "my darling boy." This was a difficult time for the whole family.

In February 2020, her apartment suffered severe water damage from a burst water pipe. My mother moved in with my brother, Mike for two weeks and my sister, Linda for one week. Darlene, Josh, Bobby, and his fiancé, April, and I worked to quickly complete the repairs. While staying with my sister she became ill and unresponsive and was taken to the hospital via ambulance. Two weeks later she was released from hospital and returned to her completely renovated apartment.

The following three weeks were the most difficult I had ever experienced in all the time she lived in my home. The once pleasant, easy-going woman constantly cried out at all hours of the night that she was dying. It was heart-wrenching to hear. She was often confused and upset. The home care workers called me down many times during the day to help with the situation. It was obvious my mother wasn't well and needed medical attention. Medical attention that neither I, my wife nor my siblings could provide.

The last time my mother went to the hospital, never to return, was one of the hardest days of my life. That day the homecare worker called me down as my mother was complaining she couldn't breathe, she was having difficulty walking and she was in complete distress. I immediately called my family to discuss with them what had been happening with our mother over the past three weeks. Most agreed she needed to go to the hospital even though Covid-19 was an issue. It was deemed her medical issues were more serious than Covid-19. This episode appeared more serious than any of her previous episodes. I called the ambulance. The paramedics arrived and they weren't able to carry my mother up the stairs in order to exit the apartment. A second ambulance was called. It took four paramedics along with me to place my mother into the ambulance.

It was Good Friday, April 10th, 2020. My mother would never return to the home she shared with me and my family for twenty-seven years. She was diagnosed with pneumonia and a bladder infection which often causes confusion in the elderly. We were told by the social worker and the head nurse she would have died if she had not gotten to the hospital. She remained there for several weeks before being admitted to a nursing home where she sadly passed away on July 28th, 2020, at ninety-one years old. COVID-19 restrictions prevented all the family from being by her side. Our sister Betty was by her side when she passed. The family takes comfort our mother wasn't completely alone when she left this earth. I dearly loved my mother and did what I thought was best for her. I hope she is not disappointed in me. My struggle with cancer has finally ended. I really do believe my mother is smiling down from heaven, happy about my good news.

However, life doesn't stop or slow down for anyone. My mother died. My brother, Wayne and his wife, Judy, died. My life-long friend Mike was fighting for his life. He'd been diagnosed with prostate cancer and gone through various treatments to no avail. He received the dreaded news that there was nothing else that could be done for him.

Mike had always stood by me in good times and in bad times. He was there for me when I got sick and I tried to help him when he was given the dreaded news he had cancer. He always had my back and I had his. He never criticized people believing no one had the right to judge another. He simply loved life. He was a great friend. He was a fabulous guitar player and an even better husband and father. We regularly got together with friends at each other's cabins. We played guitars for hours, told jokes, and consumed a few beers.

Mike thought the Beatles, the first true English rock group, were the best to ever exist. He led our guitar sessions choosing which music to perform. He included each of our favorites but made sure to slip in many Beatle tunes. Mike passed away on June 23rd, 2021, at home surrounded by his wife, daughter, and son. Josh and I had visited Mike that day and left minutes before he died. He fought the good fight always holding on to his dignity. I will always love and respect my friend. I cannot imagine how his family is coping without him.

His funeral took place during Covid-19; very few people were permitted to attend. His family asked me to be a pall bearer, an honour I will always cherish. The closing song of the service was the Beatles song "The Long and Winding Road." What an appropriate song for my best buddy. He's traveled the long and winding road of life. He'd bore his share of heartache, but never lost faith in himself, his family, or his friends. I barely kept the tears from my eyes. I truly miss my friend.

12

WHY DID I SURVIVE?

I talk about Wayne, my mother, and my best friend Mike, because they died during my battle with cancer. I was the one supposed to die yet I lived. I wasn't a better person than either of them. I wasn't an overly religious person. Didn't they deserve to live? These thoughts haunt me on a daily basis. Why do some survive and others die? I often wonder how much a person's spirit can withstand before it breaks.

In April of 2021 I have a CT scan and blood work done. The oncologist calls me at home with the result as Covid-19 restrictions prevent a face-to-face visit. She's pleased to report everything is perfect. There's no sign of cancer. She jokes that I've graduated from the Cancer Clinic and refers me back to my family doctor. It's been five years since my last chemotherapy treatment. She goes on to say that clinically, after this time period further CT scans have no medical relevance. I'm amazed, astounded, overwhelmed. I thank her for saving my life. I have indeed come from death to life. My journey of hope is complete. I sit back in the chair and shed tears of joy. I hug my wife and we both realize the journey is finally over. My sons and brothers and sisters are overjoyed with the great news. We had all fought this battle with cancer and we had all won.

December 2022, is nine years since my fight to live began. I still question why I survived. I wonder what impact I had on the world. Did I make a difference? Did it matter if I lived or died? I think about all those who have died.

My spirit and resolve came dangerously close to breaking many times. Darlene and my sons Bobby and Josh didn't allow that to happen. They physically and mentally held me up. I wonder how jumping from the wharf at the cabin would have impacted their lives. I think about the health legacy I leave my boys. They'll have to be tested earlier and regularly for both prostate and bowel cancer. I explain this is a good thing. Early detection is the key to survival. My nieces and nephews are now more aware of the importance of early testing and how it can save your life. My sons have witnessed firsthand that you can survive cancer if you fight and have supports.

I confided to my oldest nephew Michael, my concern that I hadn't had much of an impact on the world. He smiled and said, "Bob, you had a positive impact on me and I'm transferring that influence on to my children. You instilled in me the value of education no matter how trivial or unimportant it may seem to a teenager at the time. Don't you think you've had a positive influence on Bobby and Josh? Look at how they refused to let you give up. They learned that resilience from you. Just as you learned it from Pop and Nan Abbott by their actions and by the life lessons they taught you."

Josh and Bobby explain that if only one person reads my story and finds the strength to fight whatever trauma facing them, isn't that important? Isn't that having an impact on the world? If someone decides to get tested because of my story, isn't that having an impact on the world? If someone reads your story and are going through a difficult time, whether it be cancer or some other illness, and find the courage to fight, isn't that having an impact on the world. Josh confirms what my nephew had stated. I'd instilled in them the will to fight when all hope seems lost, futile. Isn't that important? The knowledge gained that each cancer, each disease is different. Isn't that important? My boys tell me I've taught them to decide for yourself if you are going to fight to live.

I have gone from death to life. I have taken the journey of hope. I have decided to get busy living. I have decided to continue fighting, to stay positive. I wanted to live. I wasn't ready to die. I wasn't ready for Louis Armstrong to sing his song. If I had died it would have been on my terms and not cancer's. It wasn't an easy journey. Ten years later I still have fears that the cancer will return. I still have blood tests to monitor if the cancer has returned. The anxiety waiting for results still exist. However, the bad days that I experience these emotions are few and far between.

I live my life enjoying the small things I never used to even consider. Seize every second, evert minute, every hour, every day you're given the privilege to live. Like everyone else, I have routine ups and downs of daily living. I remember how lucky I am to enjoy the extra time I've been granted. Darlene and I take regular vacations. Josh has graduated university. Bobby was married to April on July 23rd, 2022.

Yes, the journey from death to life was hard. The fear was overwhelming and at times unbearable. The love and support I received was inspirational. Do whatever it takes to live. Don't give up especially when your mind and body begs you to do so. Stay strong during the bad days. Take your mind to that favorite place where you feel at peace. Lean on your family, friends, and God if you believe.

My wife and sons were my rock. They picked me up when I couldn't get up. They kept me alive when I just wanted to die and be at peace. Their sheer willpower kept me alive. Find your supports and lean on them. They will help you carry your burden. Find hope and hold tight to it. Find your strength. Stay strong and live. I hope my story inspires you in some way to fight and live on your terms not on the terms of the illness you are facing.

I am just an ordinary man telling my story.

GOOD LUCK.

ACKNOWLEDGMENTS

Thanks to the great doctors and excellent nurses who really cared.

Thanks to my two sons Bob Jr. and Josh. A special thanks to my wife Darlene whose love and determination gave me the will to fight for survival when all seemed hopeless. Her inner strength and love of life kept me alive.

To my mother Alice, my father Ron, my brother Wayne and my sister Joan I miss you and will always love and think of you.

Thanks to my three brothers and four sisters.

Thanks to my lifelong friend Mike, he always had my back. I miss my friend. Mike I know you fought the good fight.

Many thanks to my sister Linda, an author in her own right. She took the time to review and edit my work. I know it wasn't easy as this was the first time I have ever attempted this type of undertaking. She displayed much patience and I will be forever grateful.

ABOUT THE AUTHOR

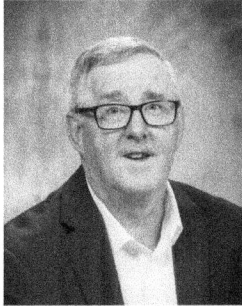

Bob retired at fifty-six years of age and one year later faced bowel, liver and lung cancer. He was given six months to live but fought back refusing to allow the cancer to dictate his fate. His wish is to instill hope to those facing the horrible battle that is cancer. To give family and friends the courage and knowledge to support them in their fight to survive.

Ten years have passed since Bob's diagnosis and he now feels physically and mentally strong enough to share his thoughts and feelings.

www.ingramcontent.com/pod-product-compliance
Lightning Source LLC
Chambersburg PA
CBHW031155020426
42333CB00013B/676